PSYCHOTHERAPY OF ANTISOCIAL BEHAVIOR AND DEPRESSION IN ADOLESCENCE

OTHER BOOKS BY RICHARD A. GARDNER

The Boys and Girls Book About Divorce

Therapeutic Communication with Children:
The Mutual Storytelling Technique

Dr. Gardner's Stories About the Real World,
Volume I

Dr. Gardner's Stories About the Real World,
Volume II

Dr. Gardner's Fairy Tales for Today's
Children

Understanding Children: A Parents Guide to
Child Rearing

MBD: The Family Book About Minimal Brain
Dysfunction

Psychotherapeutic Approaches to the
Resistant Child

Psychotherapy with Children of Divorce

Dr. Gardner's Modern Fairy Tales

The Parents Book About Divorce

The Boys and Girls Book About One-Parent
Families

The Objective Diagnosis of Minimal Brain
Dysfunction

Dorothy and the Lizard of Oz

Dr. Gardner's Fables for Our Times

The Boys and Girls Book About Stepfamilies

Family Evaluation in Child Custody
Litigation

Separation Anxiety Disorder:
Psychodynamics and Psychotherapy

Child Custody Litigation: A Guide for
Parents and Mental Health Professionals

The Psychotherapeutic Techniques of Richard
A. Gardner

Hyperactivity, the So-Called Attention-Deficit
Disorder, and the Group of MBD Syndromes

The Parental Alienation Syndrome and the
Differentiation Between Fabricated and
Genuine Child Sex Abuse

Psychotherapy with Adolescents

Family Evaluation in Child Custody
Mediation, Arbitration, and Litigation

The Girls and Boys Book About Good and
Bad Behavior

Sex Abuse Hysteria: Salem Witch Trials
Revisited

The Parents Book About Divorce–Second
Edition

The Parental Alienation Syndrome: A Guide
for Mental Health and Legal Professionals

The Psychotherapeutic Techniques of Richard
A. Gardner–Revised

Self-Esteem Problems of Children:
Psychodynamics and Psychotherapy

True and False Accusations of Child Sex
Abuse

Protocols for the Sex-Abuse Evaluation

Testifying in Court

Conduct Disorders of Childhood:
Psychodynamics and Psychotherapy

Psychogenic Learning Disabilities:
Psychodynamics and Psychotherapy

Psychotherapy with Sex-Abuse Victims: True,
False, and Hysterical Dream Analysis in
Psychotherapy

The Parental-Alienation Syndrome: A Guide
for Mental Health and Legal Professionals–
Second Edition

The Utilization of the Gardner Children's
Projective Battery

PSYCHOTHERAPY OF ANTISOCIAL BEHAVIOR AND DEPRESSION IN ADOLESCENCE

RICHARD A. GARDNER, M.D.

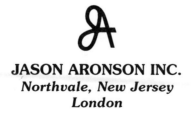

JASON ARONSON INC.
Northvale, New Jersey
London

This book was printed and bound by Book-mart Press, Inc. of North Bergen, NJ.

Copyright © 1999 by Richard A. Gardner
The hardcover edition was entitled *Psychotherapy with Adolescents*

10 9 8 7 6 5 4 3 2 1

Library of Congress Cataloging-in-Publication Data

Gardner, Richard A.
    Psychotherapy of antisocial behavior and depression in adolescence
/ Richard A. Gardner.
      p. cm.
    Originally published as part of: Psychotherapy with adolescents.
Cresskill, N.J. : Creative Therapeutics, 1988?
    Includes bibliographical references and index.
    ISBN 0–7657–0208–8 (softcover : alk. paper)
    1. Conduct disorders in adolescence—Treatment. 2. Depression in
adolescence—Treatment. 3. Adolescent psychotherapy. I. Gardner,
Richard A. Psychotherapy with adolescents. II. Title.
    [DNLM: 1. Social Behavior Disorders—in adolescence. 2. Social
Behavior Disorders—therapy. 3. Depressive Disorder—in
adolescence. 4. Depressive Disorder—therapy. 5. Psychotherapy—in
adolescence. WS 463 G223pa 1999]
RJ506.C65G373 1999
616.89'14'0835—dc21
DNLM/DLC
for Library of Congress   98–54480

Printed in the United States of America on acid-free paper. For information and catalog write to Jason Aronson Inc., 230 Livingston Street, Northvale, NJ 07647-1726, or visit our website: www.aronson.com

I dedicate this book to

My teachers at The Bronx High School of Science and Columbia College.

Their formidable influence on me during my own adolescence — as teachers, models, and mentors — has served me well throughout the course of my life.

This book represents only one small derivative of their influence.

PSYCHOTHERAPY WITH ADOLESCENTS

A Series of Books by
Richard A. Gardner

VOLUME I:
Developmental Conflicts
and Diagnostic Evaluation
in Adolescent Psychotherapy

VOLUME II:
Individual and Group Therapy
and Work with Parents
in Adolescent Psychotherapy

VOLUME III:
Psychotherapy
of Antisocial Behavior
and Depression in Adolescence

CONTENTS

ACKNOWLEDGMENTS

I wish to express my gratitude to my secretaries, Linda Gould, Carol Gibbon, and Donna La Tourette for their dedication to the typing of the manuscript of this book in its various renditions. I am indeed fortunate to have such committed assistants. I am grateful, as well, to Robert Mulholland for his astute editing of the manuscript. He did more than edit; he gave good reasons for his changes and taught me some useful grammatical principles in the course of our work together. I appreciate the contributions of Jo-Nell Long and Elizabeth Quackenbush for their careful reading of the page proofs.

My greatest debt, however, is to my adolescent patients who have taught me much over the years about the kinds of problems they can have. From their parents, as well, I have learned much that is included here. Although their names and other identifying data have been disguised, their experiences have been recorded herein. My hope is that what I have learned from them will be put to good use through this series and will contribute to the prevention and alleviation of grief and stress in others.

INTRODUCTION

Throughout the first two volumes of this series I have commented on the treatment of antisocial youngsters. One cannot write a book about adolescent treatment without mentioning them. Most therapists agree that such adolescents represent the bulk of their practices.

Accordingly, it is only fitting that I begin this third volume with details of the treatment of this important group. Although I consider adolescents *in general* to be the easiest group to work with psychotherapeutically (when one compares them to younger children and adults), the antisocial adolescent represents the exception to this principle, especially if the youngster lives in a neighborhood in which antisocial behavior is the norm. It is for this group, probably more than any other type of adolescent patient, that the combination of individual work, group therapy, and work with parents is crucial.

In Chapter Two I deal with depression, suicide, medication, and hospitalization. Although we are living at a time when most depressions are considered endogenous and therefore warrant medication as the primary treatment, I am not of this view. I recognize that I represent a small minority among psychiatrists on this point, but I still hold that the vast majority of depressions are psychogenic in etiology and are best treated psychotherapeutically. This does not preclude, however, my providing antidepressant medication as an *adjunct* to the treatment. Accordingly, when a patient comes to me who is depressed, I will ask the question: "What are you depressed about?" If the patient responds, "I really don't know," I will pursue the question further with such comments as:

> You *must* be thinking of something when you are depressed. Some bothersome thoughts must be coming into your mind. I must know what they are if I'm going to be able to help you. It can't be that your mind is a complete blank. If you think that depression has just come over you like some toxin poured over your brain, then you're probably not going to be helped much by psychotherapy, even though medication may provide *some* alleviation. It is my belief that life problems are the cause of most depressions, especially problems related to one's family, school, and job situation. The thoughts you have when you are depressed are my clues regarding how best to help you with these problems.

I consider the section on suicide to be particularly valuable in that it presents what I have found to be worthwhile criteria for differentiating between bona fide and fabricated suicidal attempts. I believe that the application of these criteria has contributed to the saving of possibly a dozen or more lives over the course of my career.

In Chapter Three I present my views on the future of the field of psychiatry—with particular emphasis on adolescent psychiatry. In recent years, although the opportunity to provide meaningful ongoing psychotherapy has been curtailed significantly by managed care programs, I still hold that there is enough value in this modality to enable it to survive and ultimately flourish.

ONE

SPECIAL CONSIDERATIONS FOR THE TREATMENT OF ANTISOCIAL BEHAVIOR

Throughout the course of this book I have made comments about adolescents' antisocial behavior. In fact, it is reasonable to state that more of this book is devoted to adolescents' antisocial behavior than to any other symptom. The primary reason for this is that antisocial behavior is the most common problem for which parents seek treatment. In this chapter I will provide elaborations of some of the points made previously. It is important to appreciate that what we refer to as antisocial behavior is very much determined by what is the norm in a particular society or cultural subgroup. For example, when I was a child attending the public schools in New York City all boys were required to wear ties. On assembly day we had to wear white shirts and red ties. A boy who refused to wear ties was considered to be "bad" and would be viewed as exhibiting antisocial behavior. High school girls at that time uniformly wore bras. If a girl refused to wear a bra during that period she might find herself expelled from school. This was not the case in the 60s and 70s and, even to a certain extent, today. A girl today, however, would be considered antisocial if she went to school wearing nothing above the waist. She might even get arrested. There are certainly cultures in which females walk around exposed in this way and are not considered atypical or antisocial. When I went to high school, if a girl were pregnant she would be expelled. There are high schools now where teen-age pregnancy is so ubiquitous that youngsters may even bring their babies to school in order to provide care for them. Last, it is important to appreciate that all children and adolescents, at times, exhibit what could be considered antisocial behavior. It is only when the antisocial acts become repetitious and consistently cause trouble that the youngster should justifiably be considered to have a psychiatric problem in this area.

FURTHER COMMENTS ON THE CAUSES OF ANTISOCIAL BEHAVIOR

At various places in this series I have discussed some of the causes of antisocial behavior. Specifically, in Vol. I (1999a) I presented a theory on the development of the capacity to experience guilt. I discussed there: 1) operative genetic-neurological factors, 2) the phenomenon of imprinting and its relationship to the development of antisocial behavior, and 3) the three stages in guilt development that relate to parental responses to good and bad behavior, namely, the pleasure-pain stage, the shame stage, and the guilt stage. Also in Vol. I (1999a) I discussed rebellion and strivings toward independence as normal adolescent phenomena from which symptomatic antisocial behavior may emerge. I then went on to explore situations conducive to the development of psychopathology in adolescence, I focused on social, cultural, and educational factors that could contribute to adolescent antisocial behavior. Specifically, I focused on day-care centers, socioeconomic deprivation, school systems, television and movies, and the legal system. I also discussed the relationship between antisocial behavior and parental deprivation of affection, identification with pathological parental traits, and parental sanction of antisocial behavior. Readers who have not read this material would do well to do so if they are to understand fully the material I present in this chapter. This material is best viewed as an extension and elaboration of that which has been presented previously, with specific focus on the previous material's relevance to the treatment of adolescents with antisocial behavior disorders.

Anger

Anger is the basic emotion with which antisocial youngsters are dealing. Fight and flight reactions are necessary for survival. When an animal is confronted with a threat to its life it generally does one of two things: it either fights or flees. Anger is the emotion attendant to the fight reaction; fear is the emotion attendant to the flight reaction. Anger has survival value in that it enhances our capacity to deal with irritations and dangers. We fight harder and more effectively when we are angry. Anger builds up when there is frustration and helplessness, and it is reduced when the irritants are removed. However, when the noxious stimulus remains, the anger persists and may even increase—resulting in even stronger emotional reactions. When there is a prolonged sense of impotence over the failure to remove a noxious stimulus, *rage* results. The difference between rage and anger is that anger is generally rational, but in the state of rage behavior becomes irrational in the service of removing the noxious stimulus. In mild irritation and anger one can still focus on the irritant and make reasonable attempts to remove it. However, with prolonged frustration and the rage that results, the anger reaction will neither be coordinated nor directed toward a specific goal. Rather, the reaction will be chaotic and therefore less likely to be effective. Even when rage is effective in removing the irritant, there are untoward side effects after its utilization. There are still "pieces to be picked up."

The term *fury* is sometimes used to describe a degree of rage that is so great that the inappropriate reactions reach insane proportions. In rage, the reaction, although inappropriate, would still not generally be considered crazy. In the state of fury, one may even commit murder—so deranging is the rage. In the state of fury the anger has reached a point where acts of violence may be repeated without reason, as if they have a life of their own. A murderer stabs the victim once or twice, but does not stop there. He or she may continue stabbing 20, 30, or 40 times. Obviously, after the first few stabs, it is likely that the victim is dead and subsequent thrusts of the knife into the body serve no further purpose. The anger has "gotten out of control" and almost has a life of its own. This is just one of the kinds of derangement that one sees in the fury reaction. Youngsters with antisocial behavior are generally suffering with frustration—frustration that has not been dealt with properly in its early phases. Accordingly, the resultant anger escalates into the phases of rage and fury and the patient thereby exhibits a wide variety of inappropriate, injudicious, and unhealthy ways of dealing with irritations and frustrations.

TYPES OF ANTISOCIAL BEHAVIOR

I divide antisocial behavior into five categories: social or gang, neurotic, psychopathic, borderline or psychotic, and antisocial behavior in the learning disabled. This is an elaboration of R.J. Marshall's four categories (1979). Although the reader may be able to identify youngsters with antisocial behavior who do not fall into one of these five categories, I consider such exceptions to be rare.

Social or Gang Delinquency

Youngsters in this category often (but certainly not always) come from homes in which they have grown up in an atmosphere of socioeconomic deprivation. As described in Vol. I (1999a), these youngsters live in constant frustration over the disparity between their own lives and those of others who are more economically sufficient or affluent. Their watching TV only intensifies their pain as they compare that which they have with that which others have (or seemingly have). The frustration and resentment they suffer build up into rage and even fury and contribute to their acting out their anger against those who they may consider to be much more fortunate than themselves. They gain support from gangs and others in the same situation. The mob has a strength greater than that of each of its individuals and this gives each member much greater power than he or she would have alone. In addition, there may be parental sanction for the gang's antisocial behavior. The parents recognize that if they themselves act out their anger against those who they consider to be more fortunate in society, they may suffer significant repercussions. Their adolescent youngsters, however, have poorer judgment and usually suffer with delusions of invulnerability. They thereby become willing candidates to act out their parental hostility because they do not really believe that they themselves will suffer. The group enhances the delusions of invulnerability in that each individual can feel even more protected by the belief that if there are to be any dangerous repercussions those around them are more likely to be affected.

I made reference in Vol. I (1999a) to studies that indicate that antisocial behavior is much more likely to be present in children who have grown up without fathers. In our society the father figure, much more than the mother, appears to be the model for a strong superego as well as the work ethic. I believe that one of the important reasons for the high delinquency rate among inner-city black ghetto children is the absence of a significant father figure in the home. There is hardly a day that passes that we do not see on television or read in the newspapers the plight of the blacks in our society and the various indignities they have suffered over the years. Although much attention has been given to a wide variety of social, cultural, economic, and psychological remedies, I do not believe that enough attention has been given to the absentee father. In the last ten years we have seen the influx of many ethnic groups into this country, a massive wave of immigration from countries all over the earth. This has been especially the case for Chinese, Japanese, Indians, Vietnamese, and Koreans. It is reasonable to state that these groups have done quite well for themselves, both educationally and economically. There is no question that they are moving into many niches in our society that could have been filled by blacks. However, the blacks have not filled these niches, even though programs have been developed to ease their entry and progress.

I believe *one* of the important factors that explains this unfortunate phenomenon relates to the absence of an adult male role model. In all of these other groups there is generally a very tight family structure with father, mother, siblings and extended family involved deeply in the children's upbringing. The fathers not only serve as models for socially acceptable behavior, but for the work ethic, educational commitment, and (in many cases) business acumen. This is not the experience for the vast majority of black children. In New York City, during the 1960s, many of the stores in Harlem were owned by white people (especially Jews). The blacks considered themselves to have been exploited by these entrepreneurs and sometimes literally burned down their stores and drove them out. Thereafter, the U.S. government provided generous and ample small-business loans to encourage blacks to enter into their own businesses. Yet, more than 20 years later, in these same areas, one finds that most of the stores are not owned by blacks. Rather they are owned by Vietnamese, Indians, Koreans, Chinese, some Jews, and an assortment of other ethnic groups. I believe that the main reason for this relates to the aforementioned absence of a father figure to provide for the children a model for the kinds of qualities necessary to run a small business, namely, reasonable education, commitment, punctuality (not "black man's time" but "white man's time"), and adherence to the work ethic. Blacks are not oblivious to this problem. One black comedian gave the following advice to his people (words are not accurate, the message is): "My suggestion is that you get up in the morning, take a pencil and a piece of paper, follow around an Oriental, and make notes of exactly what he does every single minute throughout the course of the day. Then you start doing the same thing."

There are certainly vicious cycles going on here. This is especially the case in the educational system. Black children, having few models for educational commitment at home, could have such models in their schools. Unfortunately, the public schools they attend only rarely provide such models. Their black teachers may have grown up in homes with a similar lack of educational and work commitment. The white teachers that such schools attract are often so disillusioned with the poor quality of the educational program, or so uncommitted to it, that they only "go through the motions" of teaching and thereby do not serve as good models. The teachers may merely put in their time while spending most of that time vigilant to the dangers they are exposed to in the schools. The few who are committed are so rare that they do not have a significant effect on the total system. Furthermore, many of the teachers are products of a psychopathic society in which there is a psychopathic educational system, and so they have little meaningful involvement in the educational process.

For many youngsters, both in and out of the ghettos, antisocial behavior can serve to fill up the emptiness of their lives. Hanging around on street corners can be quite boring. Antisocial behavior provides excitement. It also gets attention, even if from the police. For most youngsters, if the choice is between being ignored and getting negative or painful attention, the latter is generally preferable. There is adventure in trying to escape from the police. It is well known that drug abuse is epidemic in inner-city ghettos. Drugs serve to desensitize these youngsters to the hopelessness of their plight and provide them with some pleasure in compensation for the pains and privations they suffer daily. Having developed few if any skills by the time they reach their teens, either in the educational or extra-educational realm, they gravitate toward drugs as a narcotic to deaden their psychological pain. Drugs also serve as a tranquilizer to reduce the tensions and anxieties they feel, and as an euphoriant to compensate for their depressed feelings. Drugs, of course, can be used in group situations or in isolation. When used with others, drugs can lessen the sense of alienation and self-loathing that the drug abuser may feel. But drugs cost money, and the average adolescent is not in a position to independently afford to pay for them. Delinquency and crime provide the quickest route to supporting the drug habit.

Adolescents in the group-delinquent category are not likely to be good candidates for psychotherapy. Their problems are far more broad and extensive than can reasonably be dealt with in individual therapy, family therapy, or even group therapy (in many cases). Rather, the social and economic problems that have contributed to the development of their difficulties must be dealt with. However, even if these were dealt with at the present time, in some magic way, it probably will not do the present-day adolescents very much good. They have already been too scarred (even though only in their teens) to hope for significant cure or even amelioration of their problems. They have already been deprived of a father figure for 15 years or so. Accordingly, their chance of rectifying such a formidable defect is small. In addition, the scarring they have suffered in association with prejudice and their other privations may be so deep-seated that it is lifelong. We therapists do well not to exhibit manifestations of what I have referred to elsewhere in this book as *The Statue of Liberty syndrome*. We would also do well to heed the aforementioned ancient advice to differentiate between the things we can control and those we cannot and not try to change that which is uncontrollable. We certainly cannot control the socioeconomic factors that contribute to group delinquency while sitting in our offices doing individual therapy. Any efforts we may wish to make toward changing the situation must go far beyond that venue.

Neurotic Delinquency

I use the term neurotic delinquency to refer to neurotic behavior which is the result of maladaptive ways of dealing with intrapsychic conflicts. Here I am utilizing psychoanalytic concepts. For example, the youngster may be very angry at his parents because of the frustrations he suffers in association with their continual fighting. He recognizes, either consciously or unconsciously, that were he to express his resentment directly toward them he might suffer formidable painful punishments and even further rejection. He thereby displaces his anger onto teachers and school administrators—safer targets. The utilization of the displacement mechanism is the hallmark of the neurotic adaptation. Adolescents with severe dependency problems are not likely to express overtly their infantile needs and dependency cravings, lest they suffer significant rejection from their peers. After all, adolescents are supposed to be big and strong. Acting-out behavior, especially if exhibited over a long period, may ultimately result in one's being placed in a residential treatment center or even a jail. Although this may appear to be an undesirable placement from the point of view of the outsider, the youngster may secretly enjoy the incarceration because he can gratify therein his dependency cravings in a socially acceptable way. In such places one is insured food, clothing, and shelter without having to worry about a job. This can be accomplished in a socially acceptable way because, after all, everybody knows that only "tough guys" go to jail, not the jelly-fish types. And because everybody knows that prisoners hate jail the youngster can publicly profess that the experience is detestable, restricting, etc.—while enjoying dependency gratifications.

Occasionally, one will see an adolescent with a hypertrophied superego. This youngster has problems that are just the opposite of those described by A. M. Johnson (1949) in which "superego lacunae" result in deficiencies in conscience mechanisms. These youngsters have consciences that are too strong. Accordingly, they feel guilty over their unconscious impulses, especially those in the sexual and anger realms. When these impulses press for expression into conscious awareness the youngster feels guilty. By engaging in behavior that results in punishment, the adolescent can assuage his or her guilt. For such youngsters antisocial behavior may be attractive because it promises punitive repercussions. Although this mechanism is described frequently in the classical psychoanalytic literature, my experience has been that this is not a common phenomenon. I believe that the problem for most of my patients — as is the case for most people in western society today — is that they have too little guilt, not too much. Also this category of youngsters with hypertrophied superegos includes those who project their own superego dictates onto society and their parents and view them as persecutors. This may also result in their acting out anger against external authorities. Again, I have not seen this mechanism to be operative in more than a very small fraction of all delinquents that I have seen.

Psychopathic Delinquents

In this group are those delinquents who have superego deficiencies that result in impairment in their ability to feel guilt when they have caused others pain and suffering. The main deterrent to their antisocial behavior is the appreciation that they may be "caught in the act" and thereby punished. They are best understood to have suffered during infancy the kinds of deprivations described in Vol. I (1999a). Specifically, there were impairments in the formation of their initial attachment bonds resulting in compromises in the development of their internal guilt-evoking mechanisms. As stated in Volume I, I believe that both genetic predispositions and deprivation of parental affection have generally played a role in bringing about these deficiencies in the development of conscience. It is important to appreciate that there is a continuum among individuals with regard to the presence of internalized guilt-evoking mechanisms. On the one extreme are those who exhibit practically no evidence for the presence of such mechanisms. These individuals can indeed be referred to as psychopaths. At the other end are those with extremely powerful guilt-evoking mechanisms. Such individuals might be considered to have hypertrophied superegos. Going down the continuum again toward the extreme psychopathic end are individuals with varying degrees of psychopathic traits. The greater the absence of the factors (described in Vol. I [1999a]) that contribute to the development of conscience, the greater the likelihood that the individual will exhibit psychopathic tendencies. In Volume I, I have also described other factors – such as identification with psychopathic parents and parental sanctioning of antisocial behavior – that might contribute to the development of psychopathic delinquency in adolescents.

Last, there may be some overlap between individuals who would be classified as social or gang delinquents and those who would be classified as psychopathic delinquents. In both cases the deficiency in superego development may be the same. However, in the social delinquent the likelihood is greater that the individual comes from a socioeconomically deprived group and has learned or been taught (by direct instruction or modeling) the delinquent behavior by peers in the neighborhood. Although psychopathic delinquents may very well come from such neighborhoods, they also can come from other strata of society. However, those who do come from middle- and upper-class homes do not often have their psychopathy supported and promulgated by gangs. Rather, the home and family influences have been important in the development of the psychopathy. This factor is also related to the phenomenon that youngsters who grow up in inner-city ghettos – whose families are intact – are far less likely to develop delinquent behavior. These youngsters are more likely to have caring parents, especially father figures, who serve as models for healthy development of internalized guilt-evoking mechanisms. In short, the family influences, far more than the neighborhood, are the important determinants as to whether psychopathic behavior will arise.

Borderline or Psychotic Delinquents

Youngsters in this group suffer with severe psychiatric disturbances. Sometimes a genetic loading factor may be operative in producing the psychotic behavior. Here too there may be some overlap with the social delinquent, but the category is still useful to consider as a separate item. Like most other forms of psychopathology, it is more highly represented in the socioeconomically deprived. However, one sees delinquents in this category from middle- and upper-class homes as well. In extreme cases the youngster exhibits paranoid delusions, which may be intimately related to antisocial acting out. Believing that they are persecuted, these delinquents may act out against those whom they believe are out to harm them. Their hallucinations may dictate antisocial behavior. The voices they hear may continually urge and even demand them to harm and even kill their fantasized persecutors. These individuals will show extremely poor reality testing and other manifestations of psychosis such as looseness of associations, concrete thinking, flight of ideas, deteriorated behavior, suicidal attempts, and long-standing impairment in the ability to form meaningful relationships with others. These individuals are not likely to be members of groups because of their severe interpersonal problems. Rather, they are very much loners.

Learning-Disabled Delinquents

Many of these youngsters are quite angry because they are required to suffer daily humiliation in school where they appreciate the painful disparity between their own intellectual levels and those of their peers. When they reach the teen period they often find themselves having little if any competence in major areas. They cannot feel good about themselves regarding academic achievement because of their learning disabilities. Nor have they gained a sense of accomplishment in sports and other recreational activities because of their coordination and cognitive deficits. And they have few friends because of their neurologically based social deficits as well as their gradual removal from the mainstream of life.

Accordingly, they are excellent candidates for gravitating toward antisocial groups. They are willing to pay any price for admission to such groups, even if the price be drug addiction, alcoholism, or delinquent behavior. Because of their naiveté and gullibility they make perfect followers for leaders of delinquent groups. Because they are more likely to have delusions of invulnerability than the average youngster they are more likely to involve themselves in dangerous behavior. This is the group that explains the common finding that the IQs of delinquents are lower than nondelinquents. Elsewhere (1987b) I discuss my belief that many learning-disabled children do not have a disorder per se, but are merely unlucky enough to have cognitive weaknesses that ill equip them to succeed in the educational system designed to qualify people for functioning in our higher level, industrialized, sophisticated society. These same individuals would have done quite well had they been born into an agrarian society, where their cognitive weaknesses would not be apparent and they would not thereby be exposed to ridicule and humiliation.

TREATMENT OF ANTISOCIAL ADOLESCENTS

Many of the comments made in Vol. II (1999b) are applicable to antisocial youngsters as well. However, here I focus on further techniques that may be particularly useful in the treatment of these youngsters. The treatment of delinquents is particularly difficult because of their antagonism toward the therapist. They are typically self-centered and narcissistic. They consider themselves superior to the therapist as well as other adults in the older generation. Their attitude is generally one of scornful condescension. They cannot allow themselves to accept the fact that they have psychiatric difficulties.

It is most important that the therapist determine which of the five categories of delinquent he or she is dealing with. It is especially important to differentiate those patients whom we can help from those whom we cannot. Adolescents in the psychopathic delinquency group are not often candidates for meaningful therapy. One should try to ascertain whether the youngster has ever related to any significant figure in his or her life. If there is no such history then it is not likely that the patient will now relate—for the first time—to the examiner. Under these circumstances, the therapist does well to save everyone significant time and trouble at the outset by not embarking on a treatment program. In Vol. I (1999a) I described those youngsters with psychopathic traits which render them poor candidates for therapy. Their impairments in the ability to form relationships with others are so severe that they are not going to have the kind of foundation crucial to successful psychotherapy. With no past experience in forming psychological bonds with any other human being, it is not likely that the therapist is going to be the first exception to this pattern.

The Contributions of August Aichorn

August Aichorn was a Viennese schoolmaster who attempted to apply Freudian psychoanalytic techniques to the treatment of delinquent boys. In his classic *Wayward Youth* (1925) he described the difficulties that arose in such boys' psychiatric treatment because they were very defiant of authority and tended to see him as just another authority against whom to rebel. Aichorn was quite "street smart" and could readily identify with delinquent youngsters. He could easily talk their language and this capacity served as a catalyst for the development of a relationship with them. His basic respect for delinquents and his ability to empathize and sympathize with them played an important role in his capacity to form relationships with them. In the early phase of treatment, he would often gain their confidence by demonstrating that he was even more knowledgeable than they about crime. This resulted in their admiring and respecting him and entrenched thereby the therapeutic relationship. He even joined them in their criticism of society and its flaws. Once such a relationship was established, however, Aichorn gradually shifted his position and then attempted to foster stronger superegos in these youngsters. His hope was that their desire to maintain their relationship with him would motivate them to follow along as he encouraged and became a model for socially sanctioned behavior. His hope was that he would thereby create a neurotic, intrapsychic conflict in these youngsters, which would then be amenable to psychoanalytic treatment.

As an obvious duplicity is involved in such an approach, I would not be comfortable utilizing it. I also would have difficulty with this method because I do not consider myself particularly "street smart." However, I utilize a somewhat modified aspect of

Aichorn's method. Specifically, I do try to gain delinquents' respect by not allowing them to manipulate or deceive me. For example, if such a youngster were to start flattering me, obviously in the service of gaining some particular personal advantage, I might say: "What do you hope to gain by such flattery? It's obvious to me, and anyone who could hear you now, that you have absolutely no conviction for these compliments." By not allowing myself to be exploited I might thereby gain the respect of the psychopathic youngster. Like Aichorn, I can certainly use profanity quite freely, and I am generally far superior to these youngsters with regard to my repertoire of low-level jokes. In this way, I might also instill some admiration in the delinquent teenager.

Another complication of Aichorn's approach—and one that he does not describe in his book—relates to the fact that youngsters continually were admitted to and discharged from his facility. Under these circumstances it is easy to imagine how an "old-timer" might say to a "newcomer": "You're new here so you're probably impressed with his facade of being one of the guys. You just wait awhile, you'll see he'll change his tactics. He'll soon go into phase two in which he'll try to get you to feel guilty about what you've done." Although the old-timer may not be as articulate as the theoretical youngster just quoted, I believe that the basic appreciation of what was going on must have been known to the delinquents and have been communicated to each other. This, I suspect, must have compromised the efficacy of Aichorn's work. The approach, if one were to utilize it, is probably "safer" in a private practice setting where the patients have less opportunity to clue each other in on what is going on. J. S. Schimel (1974) and R. J. Marshall (1983) discuss Aichorn's work in greater detail.

Catharsis

Catharsis played an important role in Freud's earlier work. He believed that many of the young women he saw who suffered with hysterical paralysis were sexually inhibited. It was his theory that the paralyzed parts of the body were "cathected" with sexual libidinal energy that was not permitted free expression because of the patient's rigid superego dictates against sexual expression. It was the analyst's job to help such women become more comfortable with their sexual feelings. Such release was then supposed to alleviate and even cure their symptoms. So "liberated" these women no longer needed to utilize such symptoms as hysterical paraplegia to protect themselves from sexual overtures.

A more direct cathartic treatment related to the expression of pent-up feelings from earlier psychological traumas. In this aspect of the theory the individual's symptoms were derived from his or her failure to deal properly with earlier traumas. Especially needed was the opportunity to express the thoughts and feelings attendant to the trauma. Even years later, these suppressed and repressed complexes could contribute to the development and perpetuation of symptoms. The patient was encouraged to re-experience the early trauma (referred to as abreaction) and to release the bottled-up thoughts and feelings that were associated with it (catharsis). The analogy to an abscess is relevant here. The psychiatric disorder was viewed to be the result of the containment of the pathological process into a separate compartment of the psychic structure similar to the encapsulation of an abscess. The psychotherapeutic process of abreaction and catharsis was considered to be analagous to the surgeon's procedure of incision and drainage of the abscess. Although Freud subsequently came to appreciate that things were far more complex, some of his followers continued (and still continue) to view psychopathology in this somewhat simplistic manner. These practitioners are strong proponents of the view that patients should be encouraged to "let out their feelings." Like broken records they are constantly saying to their patients "What are your feelings about that?" and "Tell me your feelings."

The encounter groups of the 1960s and 1970s were very much in the spirit of this philosophy. Patients were encouraged to rant and rave about anything that bothered them, to "let it all hang out." The notion here was that such orgies of ventilation were therapeutic. I believe that such spectacles do not warrant the term therapy. What we want to do in therapy is help people get in touch with their thoughts and feelings—at the very earliest moments—and to direct them in civilized ways toward the sources of their frustration and difficulty. This should be done *before* the anger builds up to the level of rage and fury when the actions taken in association with such violent feelings are not likely to be judicious. In addition, the "let-it-all-hang-out" principle was sometimes used in the service of sadism. Such indiscriminate expression often ill equipped patients in these groups to deal more effectively with others in real life who were not committed to the same philosophy. Still there are physicians who naively subscribe to this belief and will refer patients with the message "He needs someone to talk to" or "He needs someone to let his feelings out on."

With regard to the proper therapeutic use of anger, I like to use the analogy of the tea kettle on a stove. The flames under the kettle cause the water to boil and the steam to be emitted from the spout. If a person has an anger-inhibition problem, one could symbolize it with a cork in the spout, obstructing the release of the anger (boiling water). Under such circumstances one could consider the therapist's job to be that of helping the patient remove the cork to allow the anger to be released. However, I believe this to be a somewhat oversimplified view of the therapeutic process. Removing the cork is only the first step. One still has to deal with a reduction or removal of the frustrations that are generating the anger in the first place (as symbolized by the flames). By connecting a tube from the spout to the flames under the kettle one can extinguish them. Then, there is no frustration, no noxious stimuli, and no anger generated. This is clearly a preferable therapeutic goal.

On occasion I will have an adolescent who uses the session to bombard me with a barrage of vilifications without cessation. Although there is much *Sturm und Drang,* and although it can become tiring to listen to the harangues, there is no question that I am serving, in part, as a safe target for the ventilation of the youngster's anger. I have often wondered in such situations what other functions I am serving, because the youngster voluntarily comes and voluntarily uses the session for this purpose. It is clear that I am a safe target and will not retaliate in ways that teachers, principals, and even parents might consider. At times, I suspect that such youngsters are trying to determine whether I still accept and tolerate them as human beings, in spite of the primitive barrage being directed at me. My "hanging in there" provides reassurance that they are not as vile as they may believe themselves to be. Also, my failure to react punitively may reassure them that their thoughts or feelings are not as dangerous as they might have considered them to be. Although I do not understand completely what has gone on,

I do know that therapists who work with antisocial adolescents have to have "thick skins" and a formidable degree of tolerance for such displays. However, this should not preclude the therapist's making every attempt to understand the sources of the anger and doing everything possible to help the youngster direct the irritation toward the initial source of provocation and to deal with it effectively.

Setting Limits

Children and adolescents most often want to learn what the limits are and most may need limits imposed upon them. Most try to get away with as much as they can and the therapist who does not impose limits may be contributing to the perpetuation of an adolescent's antisocial behavior. A therapist who is of the persuasion that one of the functions of treatment is to allow patients to express themselves fully, without significant interference by the therapist, has a misguided notion of his or her work. One of the purposes of therapy is to help people function better in the real world. The real world is not going to indulge antisocial patients. Rather, the real world may very well reject and even incarcerate antisocial individuals. Learning self-restriction should take place in the therapeutic atmosphere.

When I have a patient who acts out physically and from whom I may fear bodily harm, I inform the youngster at the outset that office treatment is for those who have enough control to inhibit themselves and not act out on their impulses. I let the patient know that if there is such threat to my person or property then I will seriously consider discontinuing office treatment and consider hospitalization. I do not make this statement as an empty threat. It comes from the conviction that a therapist cannot work in a setting where he or she is fearful of bodily harm. In a hospital setting there are certain protections that enable the therapist to work in a more relaxed fashion. One may say that I am threatening the patient here. I am in full agreement that I am. But life is filled with threats. If one doesn't pay one's electric bills, the electric company turns off the electricity. If one doesn't pay the telephone bill, the telephone company turns off the telephone. If one misuses one's drivers license it may be taken away. And a threat of discontinuation of treatment and consideration for hospitalization is in the same category. Although parents may have indulged antisocial behavior and not provided proper and reasonable consequences, this does not mean that the therapist is going to make the same mistake. I have mentioned previously the three-button panel that I have near my seat (fire, police, and medical emergency). I have on a couple of occasions pointed to the buttons, informed the patient that they are functional and have found it useful. Fortunately I have not had to use these buttons to date.

Important Themes to Focus On

It is crucial that the therapist ascertain the main sources of the youngster's anger. The primary purpose of the extended evaluation (Volume I) is to ascertain what these factors are and were. The therapist does well to differentiate between contributory factors from outside the home and those from within the home. Such a distinction is important because the therapist is not likely to get very far with the patient if there is extensive focus on the extra-familial factors. Some insight into these contributions is certainly warranted; however, there is little if anything that the therapist can do about these factors from the office setting. I am not suggesting that therapists remove themselves entirely from these extra-familial issues. In fact, they may even wish to devote themselves to changing these environmental factors, and this is certainly a noble and lofty endeavor. I am only stating that such changes involve what may be lifelong efforts and there may be little immediate change brought about by such endeavors. In the office we have to direct our efforts toward changing those things that we *can* (or hope to) change within the patient and family. Because each situation is different, I will present here some of the common themes that come up in individual sessions with antisocial adolescents.

Vengeance   Often the antisocial acting out is a way for such youngsters to wreak vengeance on parents for indignities (real or fantasized) that they may have suffered at their hands. Such youngsters have to be helped to appreciate that no matter how successful they may be in causing their parents pain and retaliation for what they themselves have suffered, they do so at their own expense. They have to be helped to appreciate that they are so blinded by their rage that they do not consider what price they themselves are paying in the service of hurting their parents. We live in a world where "getting even" is considered the macho thing to do. In contrast, standing by and allowing oneself to be subjected to occasional discomforts is often considered to be weak. The youngster has to be helped to appreciate that both sides lose in a war and most victories are Pyrrhic. For youngsters who are not familiar with the origins of the term *Pyrrhic victory* I will tell them about King Pyrrhus who lived in Greece over 2000 years ago. King Pyrrhus was obsessed with battle and drained his country's treasuries in his various conflicts. Once he fought a particularly horrible battle against the Romans at Asculum. Although he won the battle, he lost his most important officers and most of his men. At the end of the battle Pyrrhus is said to have declared, "One more such victory and I am lost." After telling this story I will try to get the youngster to relate it to his or her own situation. This is just another example of how much I prefer to rely on metaphor, allegory, parable, etc. (Volume II) in order to get across my points in the treatment of my patients.

Slavish Dependence on Peers   Another area I find useful to focus on in individual work with antisocial adolescents is that of refusing to go along with the crowd. Adolescents, their professions of independence notwithstanding, are basically sheep. The notion of being different from others will horrify most of them. They will often allow themselves to be swept up into dangerous situations rather than stand up and refuse to go along with the crowd. They have to be helped to have the courage to be truly independent, buck the tide, and not do that which, they know in their hearts, is wrong or dangerous. They have to be helped to appreciate that the person who does this is far braver than the one who blindly goes along with the crowd. Many youngsters involve themselves in smoking, drinking alcohol, and taking drugs in these kinds of situations. At the outset they basically do not particularly like these substances and may even detest them. However, in order not to be singled out as different they tolerate the discomforts attendant to their use during the initial phases. Once they have desensitized themselves to the noxious aspects of their utilization they feel good about themselves because they are now accepted by the "in" group. The next step, of course, is addiction. Then—and this may take many years—when they realize that they have been injudicious it may be too late, so addicted have they become.

I have literature which I will frequently give to adolescents describing the dangers of alcohol, marijuana and other drugs, as well as cigarette smoking. Unfortunately, these have not proved too useful. Delusions of invulnerability are generally so strong that these youngsters do not believe that they themselves can suffer the consequences of the utilization of these substances. Sometimes they are introduced into using them by a dare from some group leader and his or her followers. Such youngsters have to be helped to appreciate that it is braver to defy a dare than to submit to an injudicious one. At first the therapist may have great difficulty convincing the youngster of this obvious fact, but this should not discourage the effort.

Fight vs. Flight. Macho vs. Chickenshit   Antisocial adolescents are generally unappreciative of the judiciousness of the flight reaction. They are most often products of a society that views flight to be a sign of cowardice and fight the only proper reaction to danger. I try to help such youngsters appreciate that the flight reaction is also part of natural survival mechanisms and that all animals in the world utilize each, depending upon the situation. Both serve to preserve life. I try to impress upon the youngster that we human beings somehow have not given proper respect to the flight reaction. I believe that women in our society are much more respectful of it than men. In demonstrating the point I will often say: "When a rabbit runs away from a wolf the other animals who observe the rabbit fleeing do not generally call him 'chicken.' " I may describe the appeasement gestures found in certain lower animals. One of the best examples is the one utilized by wolves. When two wolves are fighting, they generally try to bite each other in vulnerable places—especially the neck. In the course of the fighting, at a point when it becomes apparent to both which one is going to be the victor, the animal who is on the brink of being killed will turn its neck to such a position that the area of the jugular vein and carotid artery is directly exposed to the jaws of the victorious one. This is generally referred to as an *appeasement gesture*. One would think that the victorious animal would now seize this opportunity to bite the subdued animal in the neck and end the fight instantly. However, he does no such thing. He pulls back and allows the subdued animal to escape. In fact, he cannot do otherwise. His withdrawal is locked into his genetic programming. It is a lifesaving maneuver for the subdued animal and he too has no choice but to utilize the appeasement gesture when he is on the brink of victory. I try to help the patient appreciate the importance of this maneuver, especially with regard to its lifesaving function. I emphasize that appeasement sometimes enables an individual to avoid a conflict that might result in loss of limb and even life.

In the course of my discussion I might relate to the youngster an experience I had with my son Andrew when he was about seven or eight years old. I had taken him to an amusement park. At lunch time the restaurant was quite crowded. Andrew sat down to reserve a table and I went to the counter to buy our hotdogs. There was no particular line and people were crowded about, calling out their orders to the people behind the counter. As I was standing there, it became quite clear that the young man serving hotdogs was playing a sadistic game with the customers. He was purposely avoiding giving any recognition to those who came earlier and was randomly accepting orders from the crowd. I, and a number of the other people who were trying to order, became increasingly frustrated and resentful. At one point a newcomer, who was at least three or four inches taller than I, younger, more muscular and certainly stronger, was immediately offered service by the young sadist behind the counter. The chosen one was there long enough to realize what game was being played and snickered joyfully when his request was elicited.

At that point, the anger already building up in me to a high level suddenly boiled over and I yelled to the employee: "You sadistic bastard, you know damn well that that son-of-a-bitch over there just came here...." Before I could say anything else I was confronted by the big man, red with rage, ready to lunge at me, and screaming out: "Who the hell do you think you are calling me a son-of-a-bitch? You take that back. If you don't apologize I'll beat the shit out of you." The man was ready to lunge at my neck. I had already had two hospitalizations for herniated cervical discs and I immediately recognized that the man could easily injure me for life, and possibly make me a paraplegic. But even if that were not the case, I would have responded in the same way. In a voice loud enough to make a scene that would attract as much attention as possible I responded, "Sir, you are correct! I insulted you and I had no business doing so. My apology and these people around here are all witnesses to it." At that point, the man's hands dropped to his side. There was about a 10-second silence, and he walked off and asked for his hotdogs.

I then returned to my seat and said this to Andrew: "Andrew, I want you to always remember what just happened. I hope you'll never forget what you just saw. Most fathers would not have done what I just did. Most fathers would have thought that it would be "chicken" of them to apologize to that man, especially when their sons were around. They would think that only cowards would apologize in such a situation and that they would be a poor example for their sons. I believe that I set a good example for you by what I just did. There are times when it's smart to fight, and there are other times when it's smart to run away. There are times when it's smart to apologize, and there are times when it's stupid to apologize. This was a time when it was smart to apologize. That man was wrong and he knew he was wrong. I made a mistake too. I shouldn't have called him that name. I could have thought of it all I wanted to, but it was a big mistake to say it. There are lots of crazy people in this world, and you have to be careful, or terrible things could happen to you. You know about all the trouble I've had with my neck. If that man had tried to choke me he might have broken my neck, and he might have even killed me. When I apologized I saved myself a lot of trouble, and possibly my life."

I believe that my son found this a useful experience. It may be of interest to the reader to know that I, too, found it a useful experience in that I have never again called a stranger a sadist or a son-of-a-bitch. I believe, also, that describing the experience to a patient has therapeutic benefits. It not only communicates the message of the wisdom of flight in certain situations but does so in a way that is more likely to have clout than a simple statement of the principle. Moreover, it provides an opportunity for communicating to the patient that I, too, am not perfect, I "lost my cool," and that I at times act irrationally. I thereby hope to counteract the risk that

the patient will idealize me and suffer the antitherapeutic consequences of this view.

In the context of my discussions on fight and flight I will focus
on the macho image that boys and men in our society are encouraged to assume. I will try to help the youngster appreciate that the
macho stance—especially when it has become a deep-seated personality pattern—is generally an attempt to compensate for feelings of
inadequacy. I try to help the youngster appreciate that true strength
does not have to be advertised. Of course, I am working against the
powerful influences of society, the military, the advertising industry, women who believe that macho men are more sexually potent,
and a variety of other cultural influences. These problems notwithstanding, the therapist does well to try to help antisocial youngsters
appreciate the futility and absurdity of the macho stance.

Sports   Sports can provide a healthy outlet for the antisocial
adolescent's pent-up hostility. And this value of sports can be
enjoyed at both the participant and observer levels. Like profanity,
I view sports to be one of the world's greatest inventions. Both allow
for the expression of hostility in a way that does not necessarily
cause physical harm. Although some sports expose the youngster to
the risk of such harm, the therapist should recognize that this
drawback is small compared to the formidable benefits that the
antisocial youngster may derive from involvement in competitive
sports. In Vol. I (1999a) I quoted a section from D. J. Holmes (1964)
in which he describes the salutary effects of competitive basketball
on a group of boys in a residential treatment center. The reader does
well to refer back to that extensive quotation in that it is an excellent
statement of the salubrious effects of competitive sports. I believe,
however, that there are certain competitive sports in which the
hostility element is so strong that I would not recommend them.
There is no doubt that boxing, for example, causes brain damage,
subdural hematomas, and other forms of head injury. Every year
many young men die in the ring.

I recall many years ago, while serving as a military psychiatrist,
seeing a young man of 19 who sought psychiatric consultation
because he feared he might murder someone. He was brought up in
an inner-city ghetto and spent most of his early and mid-adolescent
period in gyms, especially in training to be a boxer. When he
entered the service he did so with the understanding that he would

be allowed to involve himself primarily in boxing. This promise was kept (unusual for the service) and all was going well with him. However, about one month prior to the consultation he was informed that he was being reassigned and could no longer serve to represent his unit in boxing competitions with other units. His appeal to his superiors that they honor the original commitment made by the recruiting officer was to no avail. In subsequent weeks he found himself becoming increasingly enraged, was filled with homicidal ideation, and feared that he might kill someone. When I saw him in consultation he stated openly that he recognized that boxing protected him from murdering people and that in the ring he could let out the pent-up rage that engulfed him. Fortunately, as a physician and officer, I had more clout with his superiors than he, and I was successful in getting them to reassign this man to another unit where he could function as a boxer. I went so far to state that if this assignment was not made the man should be discharged from the military because there was a real danger that he would indeed murder someone.

I am also hesitant about football. I recognize this is an unpopular thing to say but I believe that pathological factors are operative in many (but certainly not all) of those who are committed deeply to this sport. Many antisocial patients do not readily enter into sports. Some feel like "fish out of water" when they join a team because the other youngsters speak a different language and are turned on by different things. If the therapist is successful in getting the antisocial youngster so involved he or she will be performing a valuable service.

Worthy Causes   Another vehicle for anger release that can be useful for antisocial adolescents is active participation in worthy social causes. Military service is an example of this principle, yet I am not recommending it as the first "line of defense." One of my reasons for hesitating is my belief that it is rare for military combat to be "worthy." Furthermore, recommending military service is a risky business for a therapist, especially because it may result in the youngster's being killed. Although this is an unlikely outcome of the recommendation, it must not be ignored completely. Accordingly, it is safest to make this recommendation "between wars." Also not to be ignored when making such a recommendation is the fact that military service is, without question, one of the most efficient and effective ways for antisocial individuals to act out their anger, rage, and even fury—and still enjoy social sanction for their behavior. Some are given medals for killing. In my two-year stint as an army psychiatrist I met a number of individuals who were well decorated heroes in World War II and the Korean War. Many (but certainly not all) were miserable in peacetime. The thought of war would make them joyful and I remember clearly their glee, in 1961, when the Berlin Wall was erected and we had the "good fortune" to be in Germany at the time when World War III was on the verge of breaking out. (I, in contrast, was ready to start taking antidepressant medication.)

Demonstrations in support of various worthy causes (or those that the youngster considers worthy) can also serve to release pent-up anger and reduce thereby antisocial behavior. This is especially attractive to adolescents who are rebelling anyway. Unfortunately, many antisocial adolescents are not particularly "socially minded." They are much more against society than for it, and many believe that the best thing to do with their anger is to destroy society rather than to correct it. Although channeling such antisocial youngsters' anger into these healthier directions may be difficult, the therapist should still make attempts to do so.

Dating One factor that may be operative in the antisocial boy's hostility is sexual frustration. For many of these youngsters sexual tenderness and the macho image do not fit well together. Accordingly, they deprive themselves of sexual gratification and the resulting frustration contributes to the build-up of their anger. Therapists do well to attempt to discuss girls and sex with these boys. Often, they are shy about doing so, their rough exterior notwithstanding. Sometimes group therapy can be helpful in that once in the presence of girls—especially in a situation where other boys are expressing tenderness—they may be able to let down their guard and allow themselves such displays of affection as well. If the therapist has the opportunity to speak about a situation which caused him or her some sexual excitation during adolescence, the youngster may become more comfortable expressing the sexual desires that must be present at some level.

The Talking, Feeling, and Doing Game Younger adolescents (ages 13 through 15) who may not be particularly receptive to direct talk may find useful *The Talking, Feeling, and Doing Game* (1973). There are certain cards that are particularly useful for antisocial youngsters and may serve as excellent catalysts for bringing up pertinent issues for discussion. Some examples:

What do you think about a boy who lets his dog make a mess in the house? What should his parents do?

What is one of the smartest things a person can do? Why?

What is the worst thing you can do to someone?

A girl was the only one in the class not invited to a birthday party. Why do you think she wasn't invited?

Tell about the worst mistake you ever made in your whole life.

What is the worst thing a child can say to his or her father?

Say three curse words. What do you think of people who use these words?

You accidentally break a window and you are quite sure that no one saw you do it. Tell about what you would then do.

How do you feel when you see a bully picking on someone?

What is the worst thing that ever happened to you in your whole life?

A boy came home from school with a black eye. What had happened?

Name three things that could make a person angry.

What was the worst punishment you ever got in your whole life? What had you done wrong?

How do you feel when a person with whom you are playing a game starts to cheat?

You are standing in line to buy something and a child pushes him- or herself in front of you. Show what you would do.

You are standing in line to buy something and an adult pushes him- or herself in front of you. Show what you would do.

Make believe someone grabbed something of yours. Show what you would do.

What is the most selfish thing you ever did? Make believe you are doing that thing now.

Tell about something that makes you angry. Act out what you would do if that thing were happening right now.

Make believe you are doing a bad thing.

Make believe you are smoking a cigarette. What do you think about people who smoke?

Make believe you are having an argument with someone. With whom are you arguing? What are you arguing about?

Make believe you are doing a sneaky thing.

Make believe you are playing a dirty trick on someone. What do you think about people who do that?

Make believe that you just met a bully. Show what you would do.

Group Therapy

Technical Considerations   In Vol. II (1999b) I have discussed group therapy in general. Here I comment on the specific value of group therapy in the treatment of antisocial adolescents. As mentioned, it is preferable that the antisocial youngsters be in the minority in the adolescent group. If they are in the majority then the "bad apples" are likely to spoil the good ones. In a setting in which the antisocial types are outnumbered by youngsters with other kinds of problems antisocial youngsters may come to appreciate how narrow are their repertoire of things to talk about. Those on drugs soon bore the others with their incessant repetition of the same discussions regarding the number of "trips" they have taken and the different kinds of drugs they have tried. Although those who engage in antisocial behavior such as theft, reckless driving, drunken driving sprees, etc. may have more "adventurous" material to talk about, they soon also seem repetitious to the more "straight" observers. Whereas I generally have an after-group for patients in my adult group, I do not have an after group for the adolescents. This would be especially dangerous when antisocial adolescents are in the group because they may take the after-group opportunity to exploit the straight patients in the group.

One fascinating phenomenon that I have observed in the group therapy of antisocial adolescents is the tendency of many such youngsters not to practice what they preach. On many occasions I have seen one patient tell another about the risks and drawbacks of what he or she is doing. In the sermon the listener is given traditional straight advice and encouraged to mend his or her ways. It is important for the therapist to appreciate that in order for a person to be antisocial he or she must first know what is social. Accordingly, when the therapist tells antisocial youngsters that they are being "bad" and doing the "wrong" things, he or she is not providing any new information. In fact, the therapist may be even providing cues for new forms of antisocial behavior that the youngster didn't think of previously. What may be happening when antisocial adolescent A preaches propriety to antisocial adolescent B is that A is speaking to his or her projected self and vicariously trying to bring about a change in a part of his or her own personality. The group also has the effect of impressing upon antisocial youngsters the effects of their behavior on others. Those who have greater facility with experiencing guilt and putting themselves in another person's position are likely to confront the antisocial youngsters with the effects they have on others. And this can contribute to the growth of the antisocial patient's internal guilt-evoking mechanisms. Often they do not get this feedback elsewhere because they surround themselves with other psychopathic types. In the group they are captive audience for receiving these kinds of messages.

Clinical Example   At this point I present a vignette that demonstrates well some important points regarding the group therapy of antisocial adolescents. In this particular meeting only four of the six group members were present. All four were boys. Tom, age 17, suffered with a moderately severe problem of antisocial behavior. He frequently stole from stores in which he had taken part-time jobs. He cheated on tests, stole money from his parents, and on three occasions had forged checks. He had little if any guilt or remorse over his behavior and rationalized his activities by claiming that most of his friends engaged in similar behavior. Nick, age 16, had a problem in impulse control in that he would blurt out what was on his mind without thinking about the impact on others of what he was doing or saying. He was extremely bright, but was unmotivated to do his schoolwork and so was getting poorer grades than he would otherwise have obtained. Ted, age 16, was also very bright. He came to treatment because of withdrawal from peers and difficulty making friends. He was a quiet, "uptight" youngster, who had trouble asserting himself and expressing openly his thoughts and feelings. Harry, age 15, came to treatment because of a sexual orientation problem. He found himself with both homosexual and heterosexual inclinations and, although ambivalent, entered treatment in the hope that he would go the heterosexual route. He was a strongly religious Catholic, much more religious than his parents. He was seriously thinking of entering the priesthood someday and it was clear from the outset that this career choice was, in part, made because it would protect him from any kind of sexual activity, either homo- or heterosexual.

Here I will focus on one of the group therapy sessions that was particularly useful for Tom, the boy with antisocial behavior. When the session opened Harry showed the group a copy of his school newspaper in which he was quoted. The school was a Catholic parochial school and the student body had been asked who they would choose to be if they had to be transformed into another individual. The newspaper selected what they considered to be some of the best responses. Harry's response was basically a nonresponse. In it he claimed that he was quite satisfied with himself and that he would not want to be anyone else. He focused on the fact that he was leading a good Christian life and that he was quite satisfied with how things were going for him. In the ensuing group discussion it was pointed out to Harry that his answer was basically a cop-out in that he had not really responded to the question asked of who he would choose to be if he *had* to be transformed into another person. He ignored the element in the question that *required* a transformation into *someone else*. In the service of extracting therapeutic mileage from the question, I asked Harry to try to answer the question and to try to select a specific person. I broadened it and suggested that he could choose anyone from the whole history of the world, living or dead, past or present, real or fictional. After some hesitation Harry answered: "Well, if I really had to be someone else, I would choose to be St. Anthony. He devoted himself to God and the poor. He lived in the 1200s and his parents were very rich. His parents were very resistant to his decision to become a priest. But he decided to become a monk and a priest. He gave his money to the poor and devoted his life to the poor. He went around preaching the gospels and carrying out the wishes of Jesus Christ. He lived in poverty and gave to the poor. He trusted in God in every way. He died when he was about 35. After that they made him a saint."

The other members of the group had little to say about Harry's response. Accordingly, I decided to go around the group and have each other member say which person he would choose if he had to be so transformed. Whereas in working with adults I generally would not be so structured, I will frequently utilize more directive techniques in my work with adolescents, because many of them need structure and drawing out. Accordingly, I turned to Tom and asked him the same question. His response: "I'd be H. Ross Perot. He's one of the richest guys on earth. He's got hundreds of millions of dollars. He may even be a billionaire. There's a book called *Where Eagles Dare* that tells about him. He comes from Texas. He made his money in computers. The man's a genius for making money. He owns so much of the Chevrolet company that they were scared that he would take control of the company so they bought him out."

The group had little to say about Tom's response so I turned to Ted for his answer to the question. This was Ted's response: "I would want to be Henry David Thoreau. He took two years out and lived at Walden Pond. It was very quiet and peaceful there and he got in touch with nature. He was a rugged individualist. He believed in civil disobedience if you were angry at the government and wanted to improve it."

Again there was little response to Ted's answer and so I asked Nick whom he would choose. Nick's response: "I would want to be Peter Gabriel, the rock star. He used to belong to the group *Genesis*, but then quit and has gone solo. His album *So* was a big hit last year. He gave away all of his money for worthy causes. He gave a lot of money to Amnesty International and to the World Music Organization. He gave away so much money that he went broke. So he made more records and gave more concerts and now he has more money."

Again, there was little response to Nick's answer. I then asked the group if any generalizations could be made about the four responses and whether the individuals could learn something about themselves from their answers. It became quickly apparent to all four members of the group (and myself) that all but Tom had chosen individuals who had devoted their lives to worthy causes. Harry's choice, St. Anthony, epitomized self-sacrifice for the betterment of others. Nick's choice, Peter Gabriel, was also an individual who gave unstintingly of his wealth. Ted's choice, Henry David Thoreau, was an individual who devoted himself to the betterment of mankind. When the group attempted to point out to Tom that the person he chose epitomized insatiable greed, Tom rationalized his choice by claiming that everyone wants to be rich and that all the people in the world would want to be H. Ross Perot if they could be. He was at first incredulous that the others were not committed to this value. He was dubious that the others would *really* choose to be individuals who were so self-abnegating. Having associated primarily with peers who were similarly psychopathic, he found it hard to believe that the rest of the world was not like this. Although Tom was clearly upset by the group's confrontations, I did not have the feeling that very much "sunk in," even though we spent about a half-hour on his response.

Near the end of the group meeting Harry asked me whom I would choose to be if I had to be so transformed. Were this an adult group I probably would have hesitated because the patients were not there to analyze me but to analyze themselves. For the adolescent group, however—where the emulation-identification element is quite important in treatment—I decided to answer the question. My response: "If I had to be changed, I would want to be Thomas Alva Edison. He's always been a hero of mine. He was a poor boy who through dint of hard work throughout the course of his life made many valuable contributions to mankind. And these were not only things that gave pleasure, like the phonograph record and the moving picture camera, but things that also helped save lives. For example, prior to the invention of the electric light it was very difficult to perform operations on people. Candlelight was hardly adequate, even many candles. They would often have to do operations out in the open at midday, often on rooftops. Obviously, if clouds came over or if it started to rain then things got fouled up. Also, there was a greater chance of infection." The group did not dwell long on my response, but my suspicion is that some seeds were planted regarding the work ethic and contributions to society.

In Tom's ensuing individual session we went over the points made in the group session more carefully. I repeated what I had said many times over with regard to Tom's rationalization that everyone else in the world shared his values. I granted that there were millions who did indeed view multimillionaires as being extra-special people, worthy of our emulation and admiration. But I also impressed upon him that there were millions of others—including people like Nick, Ted, and Harry—who were not in particular admiration of those who were wealthy and did not see money as an end in itself. I informed him that I considered obsessive materialism and exhibitionistic consumption to be psychiatric disorders, that is, a disease. When a disease becomes widespread, it is still a disease. When polio is epidemic it is still a disease. AIDS is still a disease even though it has become epidemic. This point was particularly difficult for Tom to appreciate because of a lifelong worship of the dollar bill.

Although Tom's defenses against these confrontations were strong, the group session represented a kind of breakthrough for him, which was the first step toward his gaining insight into his pathological attitudes toward money. It was in a setting where he had direct experience with others of different values, others with whom he had come to form meaningful relationships, that this breakthrough was possible. Derivative discussions were divided into two categories: 1) His values, i.e. what he considered good and bad, right and wrong. His particular focus was on materialism and its futility. 2) His morals, with particular emphasis on his lack of guilt over unethical and illegal activities. In discussion on both of these areas we made frequent reference to the other three group members and the values and morals exhibited in their choices.

In Harry's private session, as well, there was a subsequent discussion of his choice, St. Anthony. I communicated to him my respect for his selection, especially with regard to the sympathy for the poor and unfortunate. However, the choice also led to a discussion of his aspirations to be a priest and its relationship to his sexual problems. At the time of the discussion Harry was involved with a girl and starting to enjoy the pleasures of sex. There was no question that these enjoyable experiences were contributing to his ambivalence about his decision to become a priest. Another relevant issue that emerged from the discussion related to St. Anthony's parents. Harry saw the similarity between St. Anthony's parents and his own in that both sets of parents were resistant to their sons' becoming priests. Harry was well aware that his parents, although Catholic, were very upset about his career decision because they recognized that it served, in part, as a vehicle for suppressing his homosexuality. This then opened up the issue of defiance and rebellion against parents as a factor in his career choice.

In Ted's individual sessions we discussed his choice of Thoreau. I complimented him on his choice because Thoreau epitomized many of the best values of humankind. Ted originally wished to emphasize Thoreau's "rugged individualism" and his civil disobedience. He spoke about how much he admired Thoreau's willingness to stand up for his opinions even if it meant going to jail. He spoke about an incident in which Thoreau, when jailed for civil disobedience, was visited by Ralph Waldo Emerson who said to Thoreau, "What are you doing in here?" Thoreau answered, "What are *you* doing *out* there?" It was clear, however, that Ted was very much the opposite of Thoreau with regard to self-assertion and forthrightness. Although he admired these qualities in Thoreau, he certainly had a long way to go in this direction. Ted did, however, recognize that his choice related to his isolation and withdrawal from people, something that Thoreau had made into an asset. In the ensuing discussion, Ted was helped to appreciate that he was trying to make an asset out of his liability, i.e., trying to view as a strength his withdrawal from others. Although Thoreau may have put this to good use, in Ted's case it was clearly a liability. Ted also mentioned in his individual session his hesitation to tell Tom how revolting he felt his choice was and how alienated he was by it. I encouraged him to speak up in the following group session not only for his own benefit (in that it would provide him with another experience in expressing himself) but for Tom's benefit as well (in that it would provide Tom with another confrontation with an individual who was not genuinely in awe of billionaires, conspicuous consumers, and those obsessed with exhibitionistic materialism).

In Nick's individual session we spoke about his choice of Peter Gabriel. I complimented him on the sensitivity to the feelings of others implied in his choice and then discussed Nick's own problems in this area. Although he stated that he would want to be a person who gave to others in a self-sacrificial fashion, out of his appreciation for their plight, Nick had to agree that he sometimes had deficiencies in this area and that the choice provided him some compensation for his own weaknesses. Nick, as might have been expected, was most forthright in his condemnation of Tom – in part because he was not sensitive to any pain or embarrassment he might cause Tom by his confrontation. But for Tom's purposes (from the therapeutic point of view) Nick's insensitivity was useful in that a more inhibited and more sensitive person would not have come forth with the critical confrontation.

The reader may have noted that I complimented Nick, Ted, and Harry on their choices, but did not compliment Tom. I am very conservative with regard to paying patients compliments. There are many therapists who consider praising patients to be an important part of treatment. There is no question that many of these go overboard and their compliments then have little value. This is especially the case when the compliments become effusive, patronizing, or condescending. A rare but well-focused compliment is likely to have significant clout and thereby genuinely contribute to enhancement of the patient's self-esteem. Low self-esteem is one of the central factors contributing to the development of psychogenic psychopathology. Anything the therapist can do to enhance a patient's self-worth is likely to be therapeutic. Even though the compliment may not directly relate to the patient's symptoms it will still be useful, because enhanced self-worth of any kind will contribute to the erosion of the factors at the foundation of the symptomatology.

Behavior Modification

In Chapter Fourteen, in the section on hospitalization of antisocial acting-out patients, I will discuss in detail my views on behavior modification as a treatment modality for psychopathic youngsters. I refer the reader to that section for a full statement of my views on that issue. Here I will focus on a few important points. Although behavior modification techniques may be useful for the treatment of phobias, and various types of anxiety and panic states, I believe that such an approach can intensify antisocial behavior. My main reason for this view is that when utilized in its pure form (without meaningful and ongoing concomitant psychotherapy) it does not direct its attention to the creation of inner controls based on morals and guilt; rather, it focuses on avoidance of external punishment as a way of modifying behavior. Under the controlled situation of a behavior modification program—especially one administered in a hospital—the patient may very well appear to improve because the punishments are predictably going to be given. However, once out of the controlled situation the patient is likely to "bounce back" and exhibit psychopathic behavior because the monitors providing 24-hour vigils of the patient are no longer present. Because the treatment program had not directed itself primarily to the development of inner controls, monitored by inner feelings of guilt and shame, the individual is not likely to maintain the ostensible improvement.

ADVISING PARENTS OF ANTISOCIAL YOUNGSTERS

The Therapist's Relationship with the Parents

It behooves the therapist to do everything possible to establish a good relationship with both parents of the antisocial adolescent. And this holds regardless of the marital status of the parents. Although this principle is applicable to all children in therapy, it is even more crucial in work with antisocial adolescents. When treating youngsters with other disorders, a compromise in the relationship with the parents (if not too serious) may still allow for successful individual psychotherapy with the youngster. This is possible because one might still be able to have a reasonably good relationship with the youngster in spite of mild to moderate compromises in the parental relationships with the therapist. Because the antisocial adolescent is likely to be antagonistic to and more seriously compromised in forming a relationship with the therapist, involvement with the parents is more crucial if one is to be successful in the treatment of these youngsters. When one is dealing with a situation in which the youngster's involvement is seriously compromised and that of the parents is also deficient, then therapy is not likely to succeed or even commence.

In the initial and extended diagnostic evaluations (refer to

Volume I) it is important for the therapist to learn about those situations in the youngster's family and environment that may have contributed to the development of the antisocial behavior. Some of the more common situational factors have been described in detail in Volume I. These must be identified as well as possible and every attempt made to reduce or eliminate them. Sometimes the parents can change their tactics and approaches by simple counseling. The behavior is consciously controllable and the parents have been misguided regarding their approach to the problem. For example, the parents may not have made a proper differentiation between antisocial behavior that is harmless and that which is not. They may be coming down heavily on a youngster who insists upon wearing sloppy clothing, sporting an "offbeat" hairstyle, or keeping a room that resembles a pigsty. If the parents can be brought to the point of appreciating that these are innocuous forms of rebellion— and that they should be grateful that the youngster is not resorting to more dangerous forms—then they might be convinced to pull back.

There are other situations, however, in which the parents' contributions to the patient's symptoms are more deep-seated, and therefore less likely to change by simple advice, confrontation, and counseling. In such cases therapy for one or both of the parents may be warranted. The ideal situation is one in which the same therapist treats the youngster and both parents. Some psychoanalysts, especially those of classical persuasion, would view such an arrangement with horror and be unable to see any possible good coming from it. They would have no problem referring each of the two parents to two separate analysts, producing a situation in which three people are seeing three different analysts who may never speak to one another. Whatever benefits may be derived from each of these individual personal relationships (and I do not deny that there may be some), these advantages are more than outweighed by the disadvantages of such an arrangement. New subsystems are set up in the family and these are not necessarily healthy (even though genuine psychoanalysts may be members). The arrangement produces new "secrets," new rivalries and jealousies—all of which the family does not need. More important, the splitting arrangement deprives each therapist of the opportunity to observe interactions among the significant figures in the family and also deprives the youngster's therapist of first-hand information about what is going on in the parents' lives. Even in situations where the therapists communicate with one another, the information is generally not as direct, accurate, and rich as that which is to be gained from the same therapist working with all three. I recognize that there are situations in which this arrangement is not viable. The most blatant example would be one in which one of the parents is having an affair that is not known to the other. Under these circumstances, it is probably better (if not crucial) that the parents see separate therapists.

Structure and Coercion

Although adolescents usually complain that they are not given enough "freedom" and that they want their independence without noxious parental restrictions, there is another part of them that craves for parental guidelines, structure, and even coercion. As mentioned previously, many adolescents do better when they can rationalize their submissiveness by claiming to all that they have been "forced" into doing something. Many youngsters need this excuse in order to provide for themselves a face-saving excuse for "submitting" to treatment. The realities are that if an adolescent really does not want to come for therapy, there is nothing the parents can do to force it. They cannot drag the youngster bodily to treatment, and even if they were foolish enough to utilize such a maneuver, the competent therapist is not likely to attempt treatment under such circumstances. The parents might, however, use such coercive techniques as threatening to withhold allowances, "ground" the patient, etc. if he or she does not attend therapy. If the youngster is making good use of the sessions, in spite of such coercive techniques, then one might continue with such an arrangement and advise the parents that they should continue to provide such threats because the youngster needs them to justify his or her involvement. However, if the youngster submits to the threats and remains silent, or does not use the therapy in a meaningful way, then the treatment should be discontinued after a reasonable trial.

A number of years ago I had an experience with a patient that demonstrates well the need of the adolescent antisocial patient for parental restriction and threats. First, a little geography lesson will help the reader understand this clinical vignette better. I live and practice in Bergen County, in northern New Jersey. The area is basically a suburban community, northwest of Manhattan Island in New York City. The *Bergen Pines Hospital* is a central receiving hospital that includes a psychiatric ward for acute emergencies and short-term treatment. My patient, a 15-year-old girl with severe antisocial behavior problems lived in Bergen County, in one of the communities near my office. Her mother had a close friend who lived in New York City. This friend had a daughter, approximately the same age as my patient, who was also a close friend of my patient. These friends lived in mid-town Manhattan. Greenwich Village, a section of Manhattan, is located near the southern part of the island, about four miles from mid-town. So much for the geography lesson.

My patient, whom I will call Joan, was quite angry at her parents. Her father, a heavy smoker, suffered with lung cancer and, at the time of the incident to be described here, was in what could best be called the pre-terminal phase of his illness. He was only able to work a couple of hours a day but was still at home. It was clear that Joan was furious at him for "leaving her." The mother was a somewhat disorganized person who raised Joan on empty threats and inconsistent disciplinary policies. One day, after about four months of treatment, I received a telephone call from the mother who was in a state of agitation. She told me that Joan and she had had a fight and that Joan packed her bags and while leaving the house said to her: "I've had it. I'm leaving here forever. I'm never coming home again. I'm going out and I'm doing *my thing.* I'm going to do just what I want, when I want it. Sex, drugs, or anything else. I'm going to be a hippie and do my own thing. Name the drug and I'll take it. I'm going to drink and fuck everyone in sight: homosexual, heterosexual, or bisexual. If it feels good I'll do it. I'm going down to Greenwich Village where the people really know how to live." And, just before she slammed the door, she said to her mother, "And the only thing that'll get me back here is if Dr. Gardner sends out the police to take me to *Bergen Pines Hospital.*" The mother then told me that about an hour later she received a telephone call from Joan, who was then at the home of their friends in mid-town Manhattan. She informed me that Joan then said to her, "I'm just calling to tell you that if you think I've changed my mind about going down to Greenwich Village, you're wrong! So get that stupid idea out of your head. And as I said to you before, the only thing that'll get me to change my mind is if Dr. Gardner sends the police out after me to commit me to *Bergen Pines Hospital*." The mother then, still quite upset, asked me what she should do.

I asked the mother how long it had been since the telephone call. She informed me that Joan had called her only a minute previously and had hung up on her after the completion of the aforementioned message. I told the mother to call Joan back *immediately* and to tell her that if she wasn't home in two hours I, personally, would send the police to pick her up and have her committed to *Bergen Pines Hospital*. I told the mother that we should waste no time talking about my reasons for the suggestion, but to do what I said immediately and then we would talk about it subsequently. Accordingly, the mother called Joan and, not surprisingly, she was still at her friend's home. The mother conveyed to her my message and, again not surprisingly, Joan was home in about an hour. During the next couple of days she ranted on to her friends about what a cruel, sadistic animal I was and how I threatened to have her locked up, put in a straitjacket, in a padded cell, in *Bergen Pines Hospital* if she didn't come home. She told them that a person would have to be crazy to use me as a psychiatrist. (Interestingly, Joan continued to see me.) Her basic portrayal of the situation was such that her friends had to agree that she acted most judiciously under the circumstances, because not to return home would clearly have been a misguided choice. All basically agreed that it's better to suffer the indignities of returning home than to find oneself locked up in a padded cell on the psycho ward at *Bergen Pines Hospital*.

Now to explain my actions. First, I have absolutely no power to commit anyone to *Bergen Pines Hospital* (or any other hospital). I cannot say to men in white coats that they should put a particular individual in a straitjacket, drag her off against her will, and lock her in a padded cell. And I believe that at some level the patient was aware as well that I had no such authority. I speculated that as she crossed the George Washington Bridge into New York City she began to have second thoughts about her course of action. The prospect of going to Greenwich Village and involving herself in a program of drug abuse and sexual promiscuity was basically quite frightening to her. In fact, the prospect of merely roaming the streets of Greenwich Village alone was also, I suspected, a source of great anxiety to her. But a 15-year-old cannot come home crawling, and beseechingly say to her mother, "I'm sorry Mommy for what I said. I really am scared about going down to Greenwich Village and doing all those things I threatened to do. Please forgive me. Please let me come home." Three-year-olds talk that way, not 15-year-olds. Adolescents are too "mature," "grown up," and "independent" to speak that way.

But Joan had to find a face-saving way of getting home and the Dr. Gardner-will-commit-me-to-*Bergen-Pines-Hospital* scenario served this end. Accordingly, I provided her with the excuse she needed and enabled her to return home without shame or loss of self-esteem. One of the worst things I could have said would have been that I have no power to commit her and that Joan should be allowed to go to Greenwich Village and have the living experience that life there is not as joyous as she anticipated. As the reader well knows by this time, I am a strong proponent of the living experience notion as an important element in the psychotherapeutic process. However, one should not go too far with this concept. One doesn't sit by when patients are on the verge of committing suicide. Nor does one sit by and do nothing and allow people to have experiences that may prove to be extremely detrimental and may cause lifelong grief. And acquiring a sexually transmitted disease, becoming addicted to drugs, or placing oneself in a situation where one may become mugged, raped, or otherwise exploited is not the kind of living experience that patients need. In short, Joan needed guidance, structure, and coercion and in this situation both I and the mother provided it.

Related to the issue of parents' providing structure and coercion is the one of parents' clearly differentiating between those aspects of their youngsters' lives that they can control and those that they cannot. In Vol. II (1999b) I presented a lecture ("spiel") that I recommend parents provide their adolescent youngsters. This speech is especially appropriate to the antisocial adolescent in that many of the factors dealt with therein relate to these patients' problems. In essence, the speech involves the parents' making specific statements of the things that they can control (within the home) and those things that they cannot control (outside the home). They can "lay down the law" regarding what goes on in the home, who enters, what places of privacy will be respected and which ones will not, and what degree of the adolescents' antisocial behavior will be tolerated. The lecture also makes reference to some of the underlying psychodynamic factors that are operative in bringing about antisocial behavior, factors which parents and antisocial children should discuss. Therapists do well to utilize these same principles in their therapeutic work.

Changing Friends

Most (in fact, practically all) parents of my patients want quick cures. In fact, the most common reason for discontinuing treatment is disappointment over the fact that I do not provide this kind of magic. One of the manifestations of this desire for quick transformation of an adolescent's antisocial behavior is to insist that the youngster get different kinds of friends. The parents, with justification, are usually upset over the fact that their antisocial youngster is "hanging around with the wrong kinds of kids, the troublemakers, the fringe elements, etc." There is no question that an adolescent's antisocial behavior will be reinforced and intensified by antisocial peers. However, the hope that by associating with healthier youngsters the patient will thereby enjoy an alleviation of the symptoms is rarely realized. First, the unhealthy behavior originates within the child him- or herself. These internal etiological factors are the primary ones that the therapist must deal with in the treatment. Removing the youngster from the external influences, although it may be somewhat salutary, is at best going to have minimal effects. Even if one were successful in persuading the adolescent to remove him- or herself from such friends, the likelihood is that the youngster will not be able to relate well to the non-antisocial types. The youngster is likely to be "like a fish out of water" with these new peers, especially if the antisocial behavior is a longstanding pattern. Under these circumstances the adolescent is not going to have the repertoire of information to enable him or her to relate successfully to the healthier group. Each group has its own set of topics to discuss, special vocabulary, interests, etc. The adolescent youngster is not likely to be able to relate well to the more traditional youngster because of this important difference. The healthier youngster, similarly, will also be out of place in a setting in which the others are primarily antisocial.

This recognition should not preclude parents taking reasonable steps to prevent the youngster from associating with the antisocial types. I generally advise parents to decide who shall be permitted into their home and who shall not. Antisocial types should be excluded from the home with a specific statement regarding the reasons why, especially regarding the particular forms of antisocial behavior that the rejects have exhibited. This restriction does not prevent the youngster from associating with these types outside the home; however, at least the parent has taken some step to increase the likelihood that the patient will gravitate toward the healthier boys and girls. It is hoped that, over time, he or she will be able to relate more comfortably to these healthier adolescents. Of course, this is more likely to occur if the fundamental internal problems that are bringing about the antisocial behavior are being dealt with as well.

Advising Parents About Schools

Parents who can afford it may look into the issue of sending the youngster off to a special boarding school in the hope that there the patient will be removed from the noxious influences of antisocial friends. They often have the vision that the boarding school is populated by healthy, law abiding citizens who will have a good influence on their antisocial child. They fail to appreciate that this is most often not the case, that the other youngsters at the school have been sent there for similar reasons. Although I cannot deny that there are certain benefits that may be potentially derived from such schools, I also believe that placing the child in such an environment—on a 24-hour basis—runs the risk of a perpetuation of the symptomatology via ongoing contact with more antisocial types. Accordingly, I generally discourage parents from giving serious consideration to finding another school as a solution to antisocial problems. I try to get across the point that the problems lie within the youngster's head, the family, and possibly the environment at large and that changing the woodwork that surrounds the youngster is not likely to do very much good because it does not direct itself to the fundamental problems.

There is no question that one source of antisocial behavior is an educational system based on the assumption that all youngsters should be given the opportunity to go to college. Although some provision is made for switching to a noncollege preparatory track in high school, this is often viewed as a less desirable and less prestigious course. This is unfortunate. It results in many young-sters' "hanging in" on the college-preparatory track who have little inclination or motivation for a university education. And the resent-ment built up under these circumstances contributes to antisocial behavior. There are many youngsters who, at the junior-high-school level, are also clearly not "college material." Yet there is no option for movement into the noncollege-preparatory track at that level. The frustrations and resentments thereby suffered may contribute to antisocial behavior. In many European countries, and elsewhere in the world, youngsters are divided into three tracks between the ages of 9 and 11. One track does ultimately end in a university education. The lowest track involves training in a trade, training that starts at ages 9 to 11. And the middle track is somewhere in between. There is little stigma in these countries for youngsters moving along tracks two and three. Placement in one of the lower tracks does not automatically preclude switching to a higher one but, of course, the longer an individual has been in the second or third track, the more difficult it may be to switch to a higher one. And this same principle holds true for youngsters who proceed along vocational training at the high-school level. (I have discussed this situation in greater detail in Volume II.) Therapists do well to help those adolescents who would do better in a noncollege preparatory program switch into that track at the earliest possible time. They should help reduce the patient's feelings of stigmatiza-tion that may be associated with such placement and recognize that the structure of our educational system at this point is playing a role in contributing to their patients' difficulties.

One last comment about schools. Unfortunately, many schools in the United States promote youngsters almost automatically. Administrators argue that they do so in order to protect the youngster from the psychological trauma attendant to being re-tained. I believe that this is misguided benevolence, more often motivated by economic than humane considerations. After all, it costs more to keep a youngster in school 13 or 14 years than it does to educate the youngster for 12 years. What these administrators fail to appreciate is that the psychological trauma of being retained is an *acute* one; whereas the psychological trauma of being improperly advanced is a *chronic* one. The adolescent who repeats a grade must suffer a period of humiliation during the first few days or weeks of school. Generally, the youngster accommodates to the situation and enjoys the position of being at the same level with one's classmates. In contrast, the youngster who is inappropriately advanced suffers daily humiliation associated with the inability to keep up with peers and may have little hope of ever catching up. This is a source of chronic psychological trauma as the youngster sinks deeper and deeper behind and may ultimately end up a drop-out. This, I believe, is one of the common causes of youngsters' dropping out of school. I use the word "drop-out" here not simply to refer to the adolescent who leaves school entirely; I use it also to refer to those who just sit there year in and year out waiting until they are old enough to quit. And the boredom and ennui engendered in such situations can contribute to antisocial behavior. Such behavior becomes especially attractive because it provides excitement in an otherwise dull atmosphere.

I generally advise parents of antisocial youngsters to inform teachers that they would like very much for them to mark examinations strictly and provide the grade that is truly deserved. There should be no mercy passes. Fifty-five averages should not suddenly become 65 averages at the end of the year in order to allow the youngster to pass. This is misguided benevolence. If the patient has failed, he or she should be required to repeat the course in the summer session, and, if enough courses are failed, then the patient should be required to repeat the grade. To do otherwise is to set up a situation in which there is absolutely no repercussion for antisocial school behavior and this perpetuates the youngster's pathology. In addition, the boy or girl is being deprived of a proper education by being given passing grades for courses that are failed.

There are many schools which provide what they consider to be disciplinary measures, but which basically do not serve that purpose at all. For example, there are schools which respond to a youngster's antisocial behavior by giving some kind of negative feedback such as a "pink slip." One school in my area continually gives out pink slips, but absolutely nothing happens after one gets a pink slip. A child can have trunks filled with pink slips, yet there are absolutely no repercussions. I don't know what these people are thinking of when they provide them, but they can't really believe that they are providing a meaningful deterrent with such "disciplinary measures." Another school gives youngsters detentions. This involves keeping the youngster after school. For some this is indeed a punishment and it may serve as a deterrent. For others it is just the opposite. They enjoy spending the time in detention, horsing around with the the others who are detained. In addition, the detention may be a punishment for their parents who have to inconvenience themselves by coming to school for the youngster rather than having the boy or girl return home on the school bus. A situation is thereby set up to provide the youngster with a tool for gratifying further antisocial needs. The school, then, becomes party to the perpetuation of the pathology.

Use and Misuse of Lawyers

Many parents, especially those who have the financial means, reflexively engage the services of an attorney when their youngster's antisocial behavior comes to the attention of the police. Often they seek someone who has a reputation for "getting the kid off." These are people well known for their cunning and their ability to use every maneuver (legal, paralegal, and sometimes illegal) to protect the youngsters from the legally mandated punishments for their illegal acts. Legal technicalities are invoked, the credibility of witnesses is questioned, and other sleazy maneuvers are utilized in the service of protecting such youngsters from suffering the consequences of their illegal acts. Other parents "pull strings." They know someone who knows someone who knows the judge and thereby will obtain leniency and even enable the youngster to get off entirely without any consequences. I believe that these maneuvers are a disservice to the adolescents and serve to perpetuate their pathology. These maneuvers also entrench the delusions of invulnerability with which adolescents so often suffer. Once again, they have proven themselves immune to the punishments that others may be subjected to. Such a parent would do far better to request of the judge (either through a lawyer or directly) that that penalty be imposed which is reasonable and fair for the crime. It should not be overly lenient, nor should it be excessively punitive. This is the ideal approach to such youngsters' illegal behavior.

Sometimes the parents request that the therapist provide a letter to the court, again asking for leniency. Sometimes the lawyers, the hired guns who have been engaged to protect such youngsters and do everything possible to get them exonerated, request and even demand such letters. The hope here is that the court will view the youngster as a "sick kid" not responsible for his or her behavior. I not only advise parents that they are making a mistake by engaging the services of such attorneys but tell them, as well, that I will not be party to this kind of a program. I advise them that if I am to provide a letter it will basically recommend that the court impose whatever penalties are reasonable and just for that particular crime. I tell them, as well, that the kind of letter their lawyer would like—one which communicates to the court that the youngster's psychiatric difficulty compromised his or her ability to refrain from engaging in the crime—is not the kind of letter that I will write. To do so would only perpetuate and intensify the patient's pathology and thereby would not serve the goals of treatment. Not surprisingly, the parents will then change their minds and decide that I should not provide a letter. And their lawyer may consider my position inexplicable, totally at variance with the aims of the adversary system. The lawyer may never have considered—even for one second—the possibility that the adversary system may not be the best for all kinds of people under all circumstances. Elsewhere (1987a) I have discussed the drawbacks of the adversary system in detail.

Sometimes the claim that the youngster is in treatment will be used in court as a mitigating factor. Under these circumstances it is not uncommon for courts to withhold any punishment as long as the youngster remains in therapy. Although ostensibly benevolent, such a ruling is naive on the judge's part. The ruling contaminates the treatment because the youngster may then remain in therapy in order to be protected from the legal consequences of the crime, at a time when he or she may have seriously considered discontinuing the therapy. The ideal position for the judge to take is this: "You have committed X crime for which I am imposing Y punishment. If you want to go into treatment to help you understand why you have done this and to help you lessen the likelihood that you will do it again, that is fine with me. I wish you luck in your treatment and I hope it helps you not to do this again. Know this, if you come here again I will impose upon you a harsher punishment—under the provisions of the law. I will not consider your being in therapy as a mitigating factor. I will not let you use that manipulation nor will I accept a letter from any psychiatrist who naively believes he can use that excuse to protect you from the consequences of your crimes. If you were retarded, psychotic, or suffering with a bona fide physical disease of the brain I would not be talking to you this way. But since you are not suffering with any of these disorders I consider you completely capable of controlling your actions. Next case." Unfortunately, few judges talk this way—much to the disservice of adolescents with antisocial problems.

Shoplifting

A common crime engaged in by early adolescent girls is that of shoplifting. Most often, these youngsters will steal such things as perfume, scarves, and cheap jewelry. Department store owners know this well. When the parents learn about such behavior they are generally amazed. A common response will be: "I can't understand why she steals these things. Our family is quite well off. We could buy these things for her and have offered to do so. She could easily buy these things from her allowance." I believe that many of these thefts relate to the girl's belief that she is stealing something that enhances her sexual attractiveness. At some level, the girl believes that perfume purchased by her mother (an old, sexless object) is not as likely to have the same sexual allure as the same perfume that is stolen. After all, forbidden fruit is much sweeter than that which is acquired honestly. When department store owners catch such girls they generally come down hard on them and make various threats. The usual first response is to call in the parents, put the youngster's name on the store's record, and inform all concerned that the next time this happens the police will be brought in. Parents do well to respond with horror and indignation over the act. One of the worst things they can do is to react with calmness or to excuse the act as normal. They do well to add to the storekeeper's measures those of their own. Just about the worst thing they can do is to bring in one of those honcho lawyers who is going to "protect" the youngster from the consequences of her act. My experience has been that the storekeeper's warnings plus a parental fit is usually adequate to "cure" this problem. Of course, there are a wide variety of other reasons for shoplifting and it is certainly done by people who are not adolescent girls. I am only referring here to this small segment of the shoplifting population, and to the special motivation that is applicable to this age group.

Dealing With the Youngster
Who Abuses Drugs

Youngsters who abuse drugs often have little in their lives that they can point to with pride. Prior to the teen period most youngsters gain a sense of esteem from one or more areas. Some feel good about themselves because of their academic accomplishments. Others may excel in sports, theater, arts, or music. Some may also gain a sense of ego enhancement from social success. These are the three major areas of potential ego enhancement and each youngster may be accomplished in one or more of them. If, however, a youngster reaches the teen period and does not have a sense of high self-worth in at least one of these areas, then that individual is a prime candidate for abusing drugs. By the teen period it is often too late to gain a sense of high self-worth in one of these areas if one has not been doing anything about it previously. One cannot start to catch up academically if, when in the eighth grade, one is still functioning at the third-grade level. Simlarly, the youngsters who by then are local basketball stars have been practicing since age five or six. It is unreasonable to expect a 13-year-old to excel at a sport when he or she starts eight years later than the others. And the same is true for music, dance, theater, and other activities. It is not impossible to catch up, but it is exceedingly difficult. And the older the youngster the more difficult it may be. I am not simply referring to time devoted to the acquisition of a technical skill; I am referring to the whole mental set that precedes the technical dedication: an attitude of receptively, curiosity, and strong motivation to gain competence in a particular area. Nor am I claiming that youngsters who do not achieve competence in any of these three areas will automatically become addicted to drugs. I am only claiming that they will be at higher risk for such addiction. Other factors are clearly operative, but the failure to acquire competence in any of these three areas is an extremely important contributing factor.

Accordingly, parents of youngsters who abuse drugs have to be helped to appreciate what I have just said if they are to help their children. They have to do everything possible to encourage the boy or girl to pursue some area which may result in a genuine feeling of competence. This does not preclude their taking more immediate measures such as watching carefully what money the youngster is given in order to ensure that they are not providing money to support a drug habit. They should not "respect" the youngster's privacy regarding hiding illegal substances in the home. Youngsters without such hidden substances are certainly entitled to their privacy. These youngsters are not. To respect their privacy is to contribute to the perpetuation of a habit. Accordingly, the youngster must be told that at the parents' whim any drawer may be searched and any illegal substances found therein will be flushed down the toilet, burned, or otherwise disposed of so they cannot be used by the youngster. The youngster should also be advised by the parents that they will not permit them to see those "friends" who are also on drugs and who thereby serve as a bad influence for the patient. Such youngsters may believe that their drug abuse is normal because of its ubiquity among young people today. My answer to this is simple: when polio was epidemic it was still a disease.

Runaways

As is true of most phenomena, there are many categories of runaways. There are those who are actively or passively, overtly or covertly, encouraged to run away by family members. These are those whose families basically do not want them and are pleased when they suddenly disappear. These are the youngsters who will often find their ways to large cities where, even though in their early teens, they may become prostitutes. And I am not simply referring to young girls who become prostitutes for heterosexual men, but young boys who become prostitutes for homosexual men. Social workers and others who are involved in salvaging these youngsters know well the experience of calling the family and getting responses such as: "I'm glad she's a prostitute; tell her to send home some money. She'll finally be making herself useful." or "We don't know who you're talking about. We don't know her. (Telephone clicks.)" I have had practically no experience with the treatment of such youngsters.

The kinds of runaways I have had some experience with are those whose families do indeed want them and are genuinely grieved when the youngster's whereabouts are unknown. These parents are grief stricken over the prospect of the youngster's being killed, exploited, mutilated, etc. These parents are in constant touch with the police and are obsessed with learning about their child's whereabouts. They do not sleep nights, they can hardly eat, and they think of practically nothing but their runaway child. They are glued to the telephone in the hope that every call will convey to them a message about their child.

A common motive for such running away is anger. After all, putting parents through the aforementioned ordeal is a good way of torturing them.The maneuver, however, rests on the assumption that the parents really care. If they do not, then they will not respond with any particular concern and the youngster will thereby be deprived of sadistic gratification. Generally, youngsters in this category take care of themselves and ensure that nothing will happen to them. They may go to the home of a friend who hides them so that even the friend's parents are not aware that the youngster is in the home. Other such youngsters sleep in a park overnight. On occasion a neighbor will take the runaway into the home and protect the youngster from the indignities they have described themselves to be suffering at the hands of their parents. Although some of these neighbors are indeed protecting the youngers from bona fide abuses, often the abuses exist more in the mind of the child and the neighbor than in the actual home form which the child has fled. The neighbor has been duped into becoming an ally and providing support for alienation from the parents and flight from them. Without checking with the parents about the veracity of the youngster's complaint, the neighbor becomes party to the runaway scheme. On occasion I have had parents, who, when learning of the youngster's whereabouts, have called the neighbor only to be told that they agree with the child that he or she should not return. I generally advise parents to make the following statement to such good Samaritans: "Look, I am giving you 10 minutes to have that child back on my doorstep. If you don't I'm going to call the police and find out whether I can bring you up on charges of kidnapping."I have found this statement the best "cure" for such well-meaning but misguided Samaritans.

Sometimes, when a runaway returns after a long period during which his or her whereabouts have been unknown, the parents are so joyous over the child's return that no disciplinary or punitive measures are invoked. I can understand the great relief that such parents experience when the youngster returns. I can appreciate how joyous they are that their children are in good health and that nothing serious has befallen them. However, they are making a mistake when they do not invoke any punitive measures for the ordeal they have been put through. This does not preclude talking with the youngster about the complaints that resulted in the runaway. This does not preclude making attempts to change those factors that were operative in leading the youngster to the decision to flee the home. One can deal with those matters and still punish runaways in order to help them remember not to utilize this method of acting out when there are complaints. Accordingly, I advise such parents to let the youngster know about the grief they were suffering during their ordeal, their sleeplessness, loss of appetite, and obsessive fears that the child would be dead, kidnapped, mutilated, etc. They should try to communicate to the child what a horrible experience they have been through.Then, they should also tell the youngsters how happy and joyous they are about his or her return. And following that, they should advise the child of the punishment they are going to invoke for the runaway behavior. And there should be a punishment so severe that the youngster will long remember it.

Dealing with Incorrigibles

In the battle that antisocial youngsters have with their parents, the parents often consider themselves to be impotent. The realities are that they may be to a certain degree, but they may not be as weak as they sometimes believe. It is important that they maintain the upper hand and let the youngster know that there will be meaningful repercussions to his or her behavior. They can withdraw money from the youngster's account to pay for damaged property. They can refuse to cook meals, do laundry, give allowances, lend the car, carpool to dates, and thus deprive the youngster of a wide variety of services in response to the humilitation and indignities they suffer at the patient's hands.

There are situations in which these measures just do not work. Under those circumstances I generally advise parents to get information about placement outside the home. Although such placement is not easily accomplished, it still does exist. And although the steps that have to be taken in order to accomplish it may be long and arduous, going through them may still be useful. The very fact that the parents are taking such steps serves as a warning that things have gotten out of hand and that there will indeed be repercussions—if not immediately,then in the future. They do well to inform the youngster that there is not only such a thing as "child abuse" but also "parent abuse." Just as children are being inceasingly protected from being abused by their parents, parents too have every right to be protected from their children. The protection works both ways. However, the parents should not embark upon the program of exploring this option if they do not expect to follow it to its completion. Otherwise, it will merely serve as a false threat, which may be just one more empty threat like those that the parents have provided in the past. And this cannot but contribute to the perpetuation of the antisocial behavior.

In the area where I practice, the *Bergen Pines Hospital* (mentioned above in the case of Joan) has an acute observation ward for youngsters that they refer to as "incorrigible." However, parents cannot simply bring such youngsters over to the hospital and have them admitted to the closed ward. There is a step-by-step procedure and screening process. If successful, it may ultimately result in the police actually taking the youngster off to the hospital for observation. Often a week or two on the psychiatric ward at *Bergen Pines Hospital* is enough to sober the youngster up and may be more therapeutic than months and even years of therapy. The youngster is provided with the "living experience" that one cannot just go on wantonly destroying property, threatening one's parents, and indulging oneself in whims. Accordingly, the therapist does well to find out about local facilities and how they deal with such incorrigibles.

The therapist, as well, must let incorrigible youngsters know that he or she is not going to be sitting by passively and allow destructive behavior to take place in the office. If there is any danger that such youngsters may be physicaly acting out against the therapist's person or property that patient has to be firmly warned that office treatment is for those who are healthy enough to restrain themselves. The patient has to be helped to appreciate that any thought or feeling—no matter how unusual, embarrassing, destructive, sadistic, bizarre, etc.—is permitted in this office. However, the patient must be firmly told that threats of damage to the therapist's personal property will not be tolerated. Specifically, the patient should be told that office therapy is for healthier people who can restrain themselves from such acting out and if the youngster is going to place the therapist in a position of fear for his or her personal property then therapy will not be continued. The therapist cannot operate objectively under such tension. In addition, as mentioned previously, I *may* point out to the more threatening youngster my three-button panel, which is within arm's length of the seat in which I usually sit.The buttons provide me with immediate access to the police, the fire department, and emergency ambulances. I also inform such incorrigibles that I am in full support of the parents' steps to pursue the question of placement in a residential treatment center, such as *Bergen Pines Hospital*. Although this approach may seem stringent and even punitive to some readers, I believe that it is warranted in the treatment of antisocial incorrigibles. The message must be gotten across that they cannot wantonly indulge themselves in their destructive behavior without any repercussions. To have that view perpetuates their delusions of invulnerability and contributes to an intensification of their pathology.

In recent years a c ertain amount of publicity has been given to what is referred to as the "tough love" movement. Parents of antisocial youngsters have, with some justification, become dissatisfied with the seemingly more humane and benevolent approaches of psychiatrists, psychologists, and social workers. They believe that our attempts to give sympathy, empathy, and understanding to these youngsters is not in their best interests, that it is to "soft," and that firmer methods are warranted. I am basically in agreement with this criticism of the mental health professionals' approach to the antisocial youngster. I believe that we are indeed too soft and my hope is that the approaches described in this book present a more reasonable way of dealing with these youngsters, especially with regard to being somewhat more "hardnosed" than the traditional methods used by my colleagues. However, I believe that the "tough love" people go too far in the other direction. Many of these parents utilize methods that I would consider far too punitive and easily serve thereby as an outlet for their own pathological sadistic needs. I do not believe that they make proper differentiation between the harmless forms of antisocial behavior and those that are indeed dangerous. The method often involves the youngster's going to the home of another family that is part of the tough-love network. Although there may be certain merits to this decompression and change of scenery, the method requires the availability of a family willing to deal with the youngster's antics. Often this is a family that has spawned and reared one or more antisocial adolescent youngsters themselves and claims success with tough-love techniques. Accordingly, in the context of a curative program, the new family may be providing the antisocial youngster with another environment that induces the pathological behavior. The movement enjoyed a certain amount of publicity in the early 1980s and I am not aware of where it went by the mid- to late-1980s, the time of this writing.

Reporting Parents for Child Abuse

At the time of this writing we are witnessing a new phenomenon on the American scene. I am referring to the practice of reporting people for abusing children. Mothers are reporting fathers. Fathers are reporting mothers. Friends are reporting children. Children are reporting children. And neighbors are reporting neighbors. Children can use a "hotline" to report their parents, teachers, ministers, doctors, therapists (yes, therapists) and anyone else they may wish to—whether the complaint be bona fide or fabricated. And the reporter has a choice of three kinds of abuse: physical, sexual, and emotional. These complaints are received by a community agency that is authorized to conduct an immediate investigation. The investigating agencies often have easy access to courts that may quickly impose various kinds of restrictions on the accused person. On the one hand, one could argue that the growth of such facilities is a boon and that children are now being given more protection than they ever had before. On the other hand, there is no question that such "hotlines" are being abused by children, especially anti-social children. My experience has been that those community workers who respond to these calls tend to assume that the parents are indeed guilty of the accusations. Such an assumption has caused unnecessary grief to many. Many of these agencies are staffed by people with very little experience, some just fresh out of graduate school, with very naive views about the areas they are allegedly trained to deal with. Some are hardly more than adolescents themselves with residua of their own adolescent rebellious attitude toward the adult generation. They thereby blindly join with these youngsters and assume that the parents indeed have subjected them to the described abuses. In such cases therapists can provide a valuable service. Their knowledge of the family can be useful input and help protect innocent parents from significant grief. However, in situations in which there has been bona fide abuse the therapist's report may serve to alienate the parent and thereby compromise significantly the treatment.

In many (if not most) states therapists themselves are required by law to report cases of abuse to the proper agency. Whatever protection this may provide the child it can have an extremely detrimental effect on the therapy—to the point where it may destroy it entirely. As mentioned so often previously, the therapist should do everything possible to form and maintain a good relationship with both parents. Reporting a parent to the police, courts, or other community agency that might take punitive action is clearly one of the quickest ways to compromise or destroy the youngster's treatment. These laws present the therapist with a dilemma. If the patient is in treatment, disclosing the abuse represents a breach of the confidentiality and is unethical. However, not to report the abuse to the proper authorities is illegal and may result in the therapist's being punished. Therapists have been fined and even jailed for not alerting community authorities about the abuse divulgences revealed in the course of treatment. I believe that these laws are misguided. They should give therapists much greater flexibility to decide whether or not reporting is warranted. This is especially the case in situations in which there is an ongoing therapeutic relationship and the treatment indicated for the abuse is already under way. Reporting the abuse to outside authorities is likely to result in the disruption of the therapy because of the breach of confidentiality and the punitive measures administered to the perpetrators. Accordingly, the process that would represent the final recommendation after the disclosure is being destroyed by the revelation. This problem could be avoided if the statutes allowed qualified therapists to withhold disclosure in situations in which a therapeutic relationship had been established and in which the disclosure would clearly and predictably be detrimental to the ongoing therapeutic process.

The above represents my hope for change in the future. But what about now, when we have no such flexibility? Although we may work toward a change in these laws, they have not been changed yet and we have to deal with them as they are at this time (1988). My recommendation to therapists is that they have to make a choice. Some will be quite comfortable reporting the abuse, the disruption of the treatment notwithstanding. Others will withhold the information and thereby preserve the treatment. Those in the latter category must be clearly aware that they are taking a risk and that they may suffer consequences for their flaunting the law. I am not stating that they should avoid this position. I view such failure to report an example of nonviolent civil disobedience. We have models for individuals with deep commitments to the process, people like Henry Thoreau, Mohandes Gandhi, and Martin Luther King. The therapist who chooses to walk in the footsteps of these earthshakers must recognize that significant risks must be taken— risks of fines and incarceration. I myself am in full sympathy with such a position, but I am also sympathetic with those who choose to take the course of compliance. Therapists in both categories, however, should do what they can to bring about a change in these absurd laws.

DEALING WITH ANTISOCIAL BEHAVIOR
RELATED TO PREJUDICE

There are youngsters, especially members of minority groups, who are subjected to various forms of prejudice—overt and covert. The anger engendered by racial slurs, rejections, and taunting may contribute to antisocial behavior. This is especially the case for youngsters who agree with their persecutors that their heritage is indeed something to be ashamed about. When this second factor is present the youngster may try to hide his or her identity and "pass" as a member of what the youngster considers to be the more desirable group. Youngsters who are ashamed of their heritage often have parents with similar attitudes, and the therapist does well to look into such influences when such shame is present. This shame can also contribute to generalized feelings of low self-worth. When these parental influences are present, it is crucial that the therapist work with the parent as well if the problems that generate from the prejudice are to be solved. I will focus here on youngsters who do agree with their persecutors that their ethnic background is something to be ashamed of and their parents have either overtly or covertly communicated this message to the patient.

First, the therapist must interview the parents and find out exactly what their own feelings are about their ethnic background. Such inquiry will be easier if the therapist is of the same heritage as the parents. However, therapists who have any shame over their own heritage—whether it be the same or different from that of the parents—are ill-equipped to deal properly with this problem. The principle is no different from the one in which therapists who have never been married will find themselves when providing marital counseling. It is the same principle that compromises childless therapists in their psychotherapeutic work with children.

The therapist must attempt to help the parents (and by extension the youngster) appreciate that there is absolutely no good reason to consider one ethnic group superior (or inferior) to another. I often try to get across this message by using a number of vignettes. One involves asking the patients (from here on, when I use the word *patients*, I will be referring to the parents and/or the youngster) to envision a globe of the earth and imagine the various streams of migrations—both within and between continents—that have taken place over the history of the human race. They then do well to view the migrations of their own ancestors and trace these as accurately as they can, pinpointing as well as they can the various times in history when the migrations took place. I then point out to them that these migrations generally occurred because of one or more kinds of persecution: political, religious, racial, etc. The therapist might join in and trace his or her own heritage in a similar manner. It is useful to point out that it was extremely rare for the landed aristocracy to remove themselves voluntarily and unilaterally. It was generally only in response to some threat or some hope of bettering one's life situation that the migrations took place. Few sailed away in their yachts. Emphasizing this point can help the patients feel less atypical about their own heritage.

The therapist might ask the parents why they (or their fore-bears) came to the United States. Generally they will describe some kind of persecution. The family should then be asked why the United States was chosen from approximately 150 other countries on earth that could have been selected. Most often one will receive an answer related to this country as a land of opportunity, greater freedom, etc. Or the family may say that this country, with all its deficiencies, is still the best place on earth to live. The therapist does well, then, to point out that the United States did not achieve this status by pure chance; rather, there were very specific factors in our history that contributed to its enjoying this reputation. And one of these factors relates to the waves of immigrants who came here from all over the earth. Each generation had its own ethnic makeup. One could get more specific and talk about the early English, Spanish, and French settlers in the 15th through 18th centuries. The people who came here then were looking for various kinds of religious and political freedom—just like the forebears of the patient. One could then proceed into the middle 19th century and talk about Irish and German settlers and then the late 19th and early 20th centuries and describe Jewish, Italian, and Slavic immigrants. One can then move up to the late 20th century and talk about the recent influx of Asian people to the United States. All of these immigrants shared in common not only their persecutions abroad but their desire to work hard and enter into the American mainstream. Pointing out that the patient's family is part of this grand plan can help reduce feelings of inferiority.

The family should be helped to appreciate that just as one's heritage is nothing to be ashamed of, one's heritage is also nothing to be proud of. This may come as a surprising statement to many readers. I think it is important to differentiate between identity and pride. By identity I refer to the identification of our particular ethnic group and the individuals who preceded us. By pride I refer to the quality of feeling proud of something. I believe that one can feel pride over some accomplishment, especially one that was attained after great effort. However, I do not believe that the feelings of pride that one has in one's identity work particularly well. After all, nothing was done to achieve any goals here. Rather, one's ethnic identity relates merely to the way the genetic dice fell and where one's position is in the long trains of global migrations. If one had to take a test in heaven—and only the highest scorers were to be allowed to go down to earth and join a particular group—then there might be something to be proud of. Otherwise, the "assignment" has nothing to do with pride. It has something to do with *luck* in that sometimes the assignment is unlucky and sometimes lucky.

Many people try to enhance their pride in their heritage by pointing out illustrious individuals who are members of their ethnic group. This doesn't work very well in enhancing self-respect. The same group fails to point out an equal if not larger number of individuals who certainly have not distinguished themselves nor even contributed to the betterment of their people. The author is of the Jewish heritage and so I can speak with greater knowledge (and safety) of the manifestations of this problem in this particular group. Many Jewish people point with pride to famous Jews such as Albert Einstein, Sigmund Freud, Felix Mendelssohn, Baruch Spinoza, Benjamin Disraeli, Golda Meir, etc. My views are as follows: Einstein should certainly be proud of his accomplishments in that few individuals have made such formidable contributions to our knowledge of the universe. His parents have some right to be proud of their input into their son's growth and development. And some of his teachers as well. However, such pride should not extend to everyone else in his synagogue. I, personally, did absolutely nothing to contribute to Einstein's successes and therefore do not deserve any of the enhanced sense of self-worth that came his way. If I attempt to enhance my self-worth by warming myself in his glory, it will do me little good. In fact, it might do me some harm because I will be trying to bolster my self-esteem with a maneuver that is basically specious and thereby ego-debasing.

In the 1960s blacks realized that they were making a terrible error by joining with their persecutors and agreeing with them that there was something to be ashamed of in being black. Accordingly, they began to proclaim that they were *proud* to be black. Black is not ugly; "black is beautiful" they proclaimed. I see no point to all of this. It just won't work. Black is neither ugly nor beautiful. It is neither something to be proud of nor something to be ashamed of. It is just one of the various skin colors that human beings possess.

The family has to be helped to appreciate that anyone who thinks less of them because of their ethnic background has some derangement in thinking: "has a screw loose in his (her) head." In addition, if those who are persecuted believe that there is something wrong with them, then they too have derangements in their thinking and have "screws loose in their heads." Viewing the persecutor as having a defect can help the persecuted react with greater equanimity. The youngster and parents have to be helped to appreciate that there is something wrong with those who are prejudiced against them. Youngsters who retaliate in kind with ethnic slurs have to be helped to appreciate that they are lowering themselves and that they will not thereby enhance their self-worth. At times they should be helped to ignore the taunters and appreciate that they have defective thinking. If they feel compelled to respond they should be helped to do so in a way that addresses itself to the absurdity of the ethnic slur and to communicate the message that there is something strange and odd about the thinking of the persecutor—so strange and odd that the comments cannot be taken seriously.

I have found other comments and discussions to be helpful in this area. For example, I have on occasion told such families about a visit I made to Toronto in the year 1986. Up until the 1950s Toronto was generally considered to be the most English of all Canadian cities. However, since that time there has been a massive influx of a wide variety of ethnic groups. When I visited the city in 1986 I learned that each school district must provide ethnic and language classes for every minority group whose representation exceeds a specific number of youngsters. I no longer recall the specific number, but it was somewhere in the neighborhood of 25 or so. Once this point has been reached the educational system provides after-school classes in which the children are taught about the history and language of their ethnic group. Once a year there is a large festival in which all the ethnic groups participate, generally in their own clusters. But there is significant intermingling.

Many ethnic groups provide their own cultural programs. If the family has not joined one, they should be encouraged to find one in their area, especially for the youngster. Such experiences help the children feel that, although different, they are in no way inferior. The family has to be helped to appreciate that being different does not mean that one is inferior. Nor does it mean that one is superior. The family might also be helped to appreciate Hamlet's wisdom: "...there is nothing either good or bad, but thinking makes it so." If they view their skin color or facial characteristics as bad or ugly, they have to be helped to appreciate that such an attitude exists in the eye of the beholder and that there is absolutely no intrinsic quality that is either good, bad, right, wrong, beautiful, or ugly. In certain African tribes women's necks are stretched with numerous collars and their bodies are scarred. This is considered beautiful. In some societies obesity is viewed as beautiful and in others anorexia is the turn on. What probably is beautiful is the healthy human body. It is truly a marvelous creation and to be ashamed of it is certainly sad. If the therapist is successful in helping the family members develop healthier views about their heritage, the anger in the youngster should be reduced and this contribution to the antisocial acting out diminished.

CONCLUDING COMMENTS

Francois Villon, the 15th century French poet, asked us: "But where are the snows of yesteryear? (*Mais où sont les neiges d'antan?*)" I would ask, "But where are the juvenile delinquents of yesteryear?" We see gangs of 15-year-old delinquents roaming the streets, standing on street corners, and looking for trouble. But we don't see bands of

25-year-olds doing the same thing. Obviously, not all have "gone straight" or have enjoyed the benefits of therapy (individual, group, and family). So what happened? The angry kids grow up. Their adjustment improves; their anger diminishes. They gain knowledge, which enhances their self-esteem. They take jobs in which they channel their energies into constructive directions. They become less dependent on their parents and so have less to rebel against. This is not true of all delinquents. Some do end up in jail; others are homeless on the streets; others in mental hospitals; and others nonfunctioning members of society, parasites to those who may become involved with them. But these represent a minority; most outgrow their antisocial behavior. Accordingly, time is on the side of the therapist. After treating such a youngster two or three years there is a good chance that things will get better—even though the therapist's techniques may not have played any role in the improvement. I would like to believe, however, that the things we do can make a difference, especially the kinds of things I have described in this and previous chapters. The reader who is interested in further information on the etiology and treatment of adolescent antisocial behavior does well to refer to the publications of A. M. Johnson (1949), A. M. Johnson and S. A. Szurek (1952), J. S. Schimel, (1974), and R. J. Marshall (1979, 1983).

Antisocial youngsters reflect in part the behavior of their psychopathic society. As mentioned frequently throughout the course of this book, I believe that modern Western society has become increasingly psychopathic. There have been times and places in humankind's history when psychopathy was rampant. Like all things, trends fluctuate. And it may be that the general direction of the civilized people has been in the direction of diminished psychopathy. I can relate most directly, however, to my own life's experience in which I have observed a general deterioration of values in the last 20–30 years. In the course of treating antisocial youngsters it behooves the therapist to point out the manifestations of such psychopathy in the world at large. The therapist who is blind to these compromises, deteriorations of values, and erosion of morals is not likely to help antisocial youngsters to a significant degree. And the therapist who has taken on these values him- or herself (consciously or unconsciously) is going to be impaired even further in helping these youngsters. A therapeutic approach that relies heavily, if not exclusively, on behavior modification is likely to ignore these factors. Therapists with a commitment to the brief-therapy concept, who operate in therapeutic programs that are time limited, do not have proper appreciation for the importance of the therapist-patient relationship and its evolution. They are depriving their patients of the identification and emulation aspects of treatment and the opportunity to incorporate the therapist's morals and values.

Antisocial youngsters have impaired values and they need a therapeutic program in which there has been the development of a strong therapist-patient relationship. This is extremely unlikely to take place when the number of sessions provided is limited and finite and this is known to both at the outset. Therapists who are employed by HMOs and are ever concerned with the "cost effectiveness" of the services they are providing are also likely to compromise the development of this relationship. D. J. Holmes (1964) states this principle well (p. 250):

> It is appalling to see how far it is possible for theory to stray from the ordinary therapeutic forces which support the general society of healthy people. It is so easy to set aside the accumulated wisdom of centuries of cultural evolution as something which has all come about in some utterly random and purposeless fashion. In speaking of ego strengths, for example, or of reinforcing defenses, we have provided ourselves not only with useful conceptual tools but also with easy escape from examining those forces in our lives which really do the most to strengthen egos and reinforce defenses. The ideas connoted by such terms as *authority, moral standards, discipline* and *ideals* have fallen under a heavy shadow of suspicion in our specialty, as though they are all bad. It is even bad to say "bad." But an active day on the ward has a way of reminding one that there is really no such thing as a good boy, at least not in the natural state. They have to become good, just as we did.

TWO

DEPRESSION, SUICIDE, MEDICATION, AND HOSPITALIZATION

DEPRESSION

A common way of dividing depressive symptomatology is into the *endogenous* and *exogenous*. Endogenous depression refers to depressive symptomatology that arises from within. Generally, genetic predispositions are considered to be present, but internal psychological factors are also operative. Exogenous depressions are generally considered to be the result of external stresses. Psychiatrists tend to be divided with regard to the relative importance of these two factors. In the 1940s and 1950s, primarily under the influence of psychoanalysis, depression was generally viewed as arising from internal psychological conflicts. The genetic predisposition was considered to be minimal if not entirely absent. External factors were also considered to be important. In recent years, with the increasing popularity of the purely biological explanation, many psychiatrists view depression as resulting from genetic, metabolic, and biochemical abnormalities and do not pay much attention to the internal psychological factors and/or the external stresses. I consider the present shift toward the biological explanation to be unfortunate. I believe that there may be some genetic predisposition to depression, but it is small. I believe that the primary causes of depression in most (but not necessarily all) people relate to external stresses and internal psychological factors. The discussion here is based on this assumption.

I recognize that I am in the minority on this subject among my colleagues in the field of psychiatry. I have given serious consideration to new developments in the field that rely heavily on the theory of primary biological etiology, but I still hold that the weight of the evidence supports the position that adolescent depressions of the kind I discuss in this chapter are best understood as manifestations of internal psychological and environmental processes. I am not referring here to manic-depressive psychosis, in which the evidence for a biological-genetic predisposition is strong. I am referring to the much more common types of depression seen in adolescence.

Environmental Factors

With regard to the exogenous factors, it behooves the examiner to look carefully into the family and other environmental factors that may be contributing to the youngster's depression. The extensive evaluation that I described in Vol. I (1999a) can serve this purpose well. Not to conduct such an exhaustive evaluation is likely to compromise the treatment because the examiner will be deprived of learning about the environmental factors that are likely to have contributed to the depression. And this is one of my strongest criticisms of biologically oriented psychiatrists. They generally do not delve deeply enough into the details of their patients' backgrounds. Committed to the notion that depression is primarily, if not entirely, biologically derived they can justify their failure to conduct such an investigation. Subscribing to the biological theory also enables them to provide what appears to be a relatively quick and easily administered form of treatment, namely, medication. As I will discuss later in this chapter, I believe that antidepressants may be of symptomatic value in the treatment of the vast majority of depressions. But this is not inconsistent with my belief that environmental and psychological factors are the paramount etiological factors. Palliation is not the same as cure.

Accordingly, the examiner must try to ascertain what the environmental factors have been that have contributed to the depression. Perhaps the youngster has been exposed to ongoing marital conflicts, especially those that culminate in separation and/or divorce. Exposure to and/or embroilment in custody litigation is an even greater environmental trauma because the youngster cannot but feel like a rope in a tug of war. The loyalty conflicts engendered by such litigation are enormous and the likelihood that the youngster will become depressed when so embroiled is extremely high. Elsewhere (1986), I have discussed in detail the ways in which custody litigation can contribute to a wide variety of psychopathological reactions including depression. Perhaps the youngster suffers with a learning disability and thereby experiences inordinate academic stresses which can lead to depression (Gardner, 1987b). Some youngsters are likely to become depressed in their dealings with members of the opposite sex. The dating period can be extremely anxiety provoking, its gratifications notwithstanding. Rejections in this realm are a common source of depression (and even suicide) among adolescents.

Many youngsters become depressed over the socioeconomic conditions in which they have grown up. Patients used as subjects in studies of depression in childhood and adolescence often come from inner city ghettos. This is an easy population in which to find depressed children. Many adolescents growing up in such areas use drugs as their antidepressant. It is rare for such studies to derive their patients from affluent suburbs. The youngster who does poorly in sports (possibly related to genetic and/or biological weaknesses) may become depressed in an environment which is highly sports oriented. A youngster of average intelligence who grows up in a home with a sibling who is an academic "superstar" may also become depressed. The youngster who cannot live up to his or her parents' inordinately high academic standards is also likely to become depressed. I could provide many other examples. My primary point here is that the examiner should investigate every possible environmental factor that may produce depression and do whatever can be done to alter these. And such changes are most predictably accomplished when the therapist works with both the youngster and the parents.

Internal Psychological Factors

Anger Inhibition   In addition to the exogenous factors, complex internal psychological mechanisms are also often operative in bringing about depression. One factor that may contribute to depression is inhibition in the expression of anger. The person's anger becomes turned inward and directed toward oneself. The inhibition of such rage is likely to produce depressed feelings. Furthermore, individuals who are inhibited in the expression of anger may develop self-flagellatory symptomatology. They constantly castigate themselves with comments such as "I'm stupid to have done that," "What a wretch I am," and "What a fool I've been." The person may justify such self-recrimination by dwelling on past indiscretions that may have long since been forgotten. These are trivial and do not warrant the degree of self-denigration that the individual exhibits. Errors and minor indiscretions become exaggerated into heinous crimes. When self-flagellatory symptoms are present, one can generally assume that such patients are fearful of and/or guilty over directly expressing anger to others, upon whom they may be quite dependent. They therefore direct their anger toward themselves, a safer target. In working with such patients it is important to help them become less inhibited in the expression of their anger. They may have grown up in families where the parents were similarly inhibited. The parents may have boasted that they have been married many years and never had a fight. In such a marriage it is likely that one or both of the parents have anger inhibition problems. Many such inhibited youngsters may have been exposed to harsh disciplinary and punitive measures in the context of which they may have been told, "Nice boys and girls never say such things to their parents. They never even *think* such things."

Guilt   A further contributing factor to depression is guilt. By guilt I refer to the feeling of low self-worth experienced following thoughts, feelings, and acts which the individual has learned are unacceptable to significant figures in his or her environment. In essence, the guilty person is saying: "How terrible a person I am for what I have thought, felt, or done." Feelings of low self-worth attendant to guilt are likely to contribute to the depressive symptomatology. Accordingly, the examiner does well to investigate into factors that may be guilt-evoking. As mentioned, many children are often taught to feel guilty about the expression of hostility toward a parent: "How can you do this to your mother?" and "What a terrible thing to say to your father." The examiner does well to look into things that the youngster him- or herself might be doing that may engender guilty feelings. If the youngster has a healthy superego, then performing such acts as cheating, lying, and stealing may be associated with guilt. In such cases the guilt is appropriate. However, there are youngsters who suffer with inappropriate or exaggerated guilt, such as guilt over sexual feelings, masturbation, or sexual activities at an age-appropriate level (in the examiner's opinion). In such situations, it behooves the examiner to try to reduce such guilt in the service of alleviating the depressive feelings.

When working with patients who have excessive guilt, it is important for the examiner to appreciate that most patients have too little guilt, rather than too much guilt. We are living very much in a psychopathic society. There are some who work on the principle that the therapist should try always to reduce guilt and that increasing guilt cannot but be antitherapeutic. This is absurd. Most people need *more* guilt than less guilt. Accordingly, there are many situations in which the therapist must do everything possible to *increase* guilt in order to help turn the youngster from a psychopathic personality into a civilized human being, sensitive to the feelings of others. But this is an aside. My main point here is that youngsters with an inordinate degree of guilt are prone to become depressed and anything that the examiner can do to reduce guilt will thereby contribute to the alleviation of depression.

Failure to Achieve Certain Aspirations   People who are prone to become depressed are often those with three sets of aspirations that must be maintained if they are to feel worthy. When these goals are not maintained, they tend to react with depressed feelings. The three goals are: 1) the wish to be loved and respected, 2) the wish to be strong, superior, and secure, and 3) the wish to be good and loving rather than hateful and destructive. Some youngsters who are depressed have inordinate needs to be loved and respected. In response to some privations in this area they may have exaggerated needs for compensatory respect and affection. These inordinate needs and demands may result in chronic feelings of dissatisfaction. It it is the job of the therapist to help such youngsters develop more realistic goals with regard to the degree of love and respect they can reasonably hope to obtain from other human beings. Unfortunately, if they are swept up in the romantic love myth—which often promises enormous love and infinite respect—then their frustrations and disillusionment in this area are likely to be formidable.

With regard to the second set of aspirations—to be strong, superior, and secure—boys especially may experience frustration. In the macho world in which they grow up, any signs of weakness or even normal degrees of insecurity may not be tolerable. Inordinate aspirations in this realm are likely to result in the kinds of frustrations and disappointments that contribute to depression. The examiner must help such youngsters gain a more realistic view of what their potentials are and recognize that many who are seemingly stable in this respect are often presenting a facade. Such a youngster has to be helped to appreciate that even those who have exhibited genuine accomplishments still have feelings of insecurity.

With regard to the third realm—the wish to be good and loving rather than hateful and destructive—such youngsters may have the idea that there are all-loving people who do not harbor any hateful feelings at all toward anyone. They have to be helped to appreciate that all human relationships are ambivalent and that even the most loving person harbors within him- or herself deep-seated, hostile, and even hateful feelings. If the therapist is successful in convincing the youngster of the validity of this view, then aspirations may be lowered and this contributing element in depression may be reduced.

Dependency Problems Individuals who easily become depressed are often quite dependent. Not being able to function adequately at age-appropriate levels, they easily slide back into more infantile levels where they gratify their dependent needs. Of course, such individuals require the presence of caretakers who will indulge their dependency demands. Such youngsters are likely to regress to infantile states of helplessness in stressful situations when they do not feel they have the capacity to cope. At such times, depressed patients become clinging and demand support and protection from those around them. It behooves the examiner to help such youngsters deal more adequately with the stresses of life, to learn more about how to cope with reality, and thereby to deal better with stresses. Also, they have to work with the caretaking individuals who might be indulging the dependency gratifications and thereby perpetuating the depression. Sometimes, this is more easily said than done in that the caretakers may rationalize their indulgence to significant degrees. They may view the examiner who requests that they pull back and not provide such indulgences as being cruel and insensitive.

Reactions to Loss   Individuals who are depression prone are more likely to react in an exaggerated fashion to significant loss than those who do not become depressed. Sometimes the loss is realistic, such as the loss of a parent, sibling, or loved one. Sometimes the loss is symbolic in that the individual considers the loss to be greater than it really is. A good example of this would be the loss of a boyfriend or girlfriend— someone who, in reality, could be replaced much more easily than the youngster can possibly imagine. Youngsters who are in the latter category should be helped to appreciate that an important factor in the romantic love phenomenon is the projection onto the loved person of one's own aspirations about what an individual should be. In situations where the loss is more real, such as death and divorce, the youngster has to be helped to cope more adequately with these losses. Elsewhere (1983), I have provided advice to such youngsters.

Depression and the Fight/Flight Reaction   The fight/flight reactions are of survival value. When confronted with a danger, organisms at all levels either fight or flee. This is an essential mechanism for survival. Some individuals are more likely to fight when confronted with a danger and others more likely to flee. It is probable that both genetic and environmental factors contribute to the pattern that will be selected. The healthy individual is capable of making a judicious decision regarding which mechanism to bring into operation when confronted with a threat. I view many depression-prone individuals as people who are fearful of invoking either of these survival mechanisms, i.e., they are too frightened to fight because they do not view themselves as having effective weapons and they fear flight because they do not consider themselves capable of surviving independently. They need protectors at their side — not only to protect them from the threats of others but to provide for them because they do not feel themselves capable of providing for themselves. They become immobile and paralyzed in a neutral position. They neither fight nor flee. In their immobility they protect themselves from the untoward consequences they anticipate if they were to surge forward and fight the threat. In addition, their immobilization and failure to flee ensures their being protected and taken care of by their protectors.

The "success" of the depressive maneuver requires the attendance of caretaking individuals who will provide the indulgence and protection the depressive person requests, demands, or elicits. Without such individuals the reaction may not be utilized. Well-meaning figures in the depressed person's environment are often drawn into the game, not realizing that their indulgence is a disservice. They may consider themselves loving, sacrificial, giving, and devoted. Although some of those qualities are without doubt present, the caretakers often fail to appreciate that the same maneuvers are perpetuating the depressive symptomatology. Examiners who work with depressed adolescents do well to consider this important possible contribution to the youngster's depression. These young people have to be helped to assert themselves and fight more ardently when the situation warrants it and to develop greater independence so they will not become immobilized and have to rely on caretakers when exposed to external stresses and threats. And the caretaking individuals have to be helped similarly to reduce their indulgence.

Nuclear War   We frequently read in newspaper and magazine articles the theory that growing up in a nuclear age can cause young people to become unmotivated and depressed. The prospect of being annihilated in nuclear warfare is said to contribute to poor motivation, boredom, and the lack of commitment to life. And this theory has been invoked to explain teen suicide as well. Although there are certainly youngsters who concern themselves with the prospect of a nuclear holocaust, I have not seen such concern contribute to the formation of clinical symptoms—depression, suicidal attempts, or any other symptoms. Most (but certainly not all) of the youngsters I have seen in my office are not concerned significantly with such issues as politics, wars, and the possibility of a nuclear holocaust. They are much more concerned with their schools, friends, and family. When symptoms develop, they are usually derived from problems in these three areas. When one considers the adolescent's delusions of invulnerability, concerns with nuclear wars become even more remote. In fact, I would go further and say that most adolescents would believe that if there were a nuclear war, they would be among the survivors. And this is not only true regarding exposure to the initial blast, but on the remote level of suffering future consequences of radioactive fallout, burns, etc.

SUICIDE

Adolescent suicide is the second leading cause of death in the United States for individuals between the ages of 15 and 24. (Accidents are the most common cause of death in the teen period.) And the suicidal rate in this age bracket has been increasing. In 1950 the rate was 4.5 per 100,000. This increased to the point where in 1980 it was 12.3 per 100,000. During the 1980s the rate has leveled off, but is still at approximately the 12 per 100,000 range (K. Simmons, 1987a).

Some depressed patients become suicidal. It is important for examiners to appreciate that just about all human beings have suicidal thoughts at times. Life predictably produces frustrations, disappointments, and feelings of impotence. Everyone, at times, gets depressed. People will have the feeling, at times, that "it's just not worth it." Obviously, it would be impossible to obtain normative data regarding just how frequent such thoughts are. It is reasonable to speculate, however, that there is a gradation from the normal level of such thoughts to the pathological frequency. If the examiner worked under the assumption that normal healthy people *never* have such thoughts, then a much higher percentage of patients would be considered suicidal. One wants to learn about the frequency of such thoughts and, of course, the content. Content, especially, will be useful in helping the examiner differentiate between bona fide and fabricated suicidal attempts and preoccupations.

Therapists who work with adolescents may be asked to make a decision regarding whether or not a youngster who threatens suicide should be hospitalized. This is an extremely important question and the ability of the therapist to differentiate between bona fide and fabricated suicidal threats may determine whether a youngster lives or dies. Accordingly, I will present here what I consider to be important differentiating criteria between the two groups. I believe that these criteria will most often enable the therapist to make a decision regarding which category the patient is in. However, there may be occasions when the examiner is not certain. Under these circumstances it is best to err on the side of caution and to hospitalize. I will have more to say about these ambiguous situations below.

I wish to emphasize at this point the importance of the examiner's not conducting a suicide evaluation under conditions of time constraints. That the evaluation may be considered urgent does not mean that the patient need be rushed through it. It is extremely unlikely that the patient is going to try to commit suicide in the therapist's presence. Accordingly, a few hours devoted to the evaluation is reasonable to expect of both the therapist, the patient, and the family. A physician working in an emergency room is in no position to do a proper suicide evaluation. Nor is a therapist working in a clinic setting where the examiner is required to devote only a specific amount of time to each patient. Evaluators working for HMOs that are ever concerned with the "cost effectiveness" of the services provided may also be compromised in their ability to conduct an adequate evaluation for suicide. People do not tell surgeons that they must operate within a particular time frame. All appreciate the fact that the surgeon may not know exactly what to do until the patient is opened. The same principle holds for the psychiatric evaluation and is especially valid when one is considering the possibility of suicide. Evaluators do well, therefore, to refuse to conduct such examinations unless they are given the freedom to spend as much time as they consider warranted.

Bona Fide Suicidal Attempts

First, I will describe those manifestations that generally indicate serious depression. When these factors are present they increase significantly the likelihood that the suicidal threat is genuine. One wants to ascertain whether the threat is made by a youngster who is exhibiting a broader picture of moderately severe to severe depression. Some of the more common manifestations of such depression are psychomotor retardation, severe self-flagellatory and self-deprecatory statements ("I'm no good." "I deserve to die." "I'm loathesome, wretched, etc."). Statements of hopelessness about the future are common as well as profound feelings of helplessness. Patients who spontaneously and frequently speak about their belief that no one will miss them if they die may be a serious suicidal risk. This is an extremely important area to investigate. The realities may be that many close friends and relatives would suffer great grief if the youngster were to commit suicide. If, however, the patient *believes* that none of these individuals care, then the suicidal risk is enhanced formidably.

The presence of psychotic symptoms, such as hallucinations and delusions, increases the suicidal risk. Particularly dangerous are delusions in which the patient views the suicide as a method for joining dead relatives in the afterlife. Of course, if the therapist believes that one does indeed have the opportunity to join dead relatives in the afterlife, then this might not be considered a delusion. It is hoped, however, that the therapist will be of the persuasion that at the age of 16 it is somewhat early for such reconciliation and that it would be better to allow natural forces to determine when this great day of rapprochement takes place. Patients with such a delusion may also hear voices that encourage or order suicide to hasten the journey into the afterlife. Or, the psychotic youngster may respond to delusions of persecution from which the only escape is to kill oneself.

Loss of appetite, loss of sexual desire, sleeplessness, profound feelings of low self-worth, and feelings of painful boredom also enhance the suicidal risk. Other manifestations of severe depression include withdrawal from socialization, loss of interest in friends, lack of pleasure in any activity, weeping episodes, flat depressive affect, and inhibition in expressing anger. In fact, the inhibition in expressing anger may contribute to the aforementioned self-flagel-latory statements.

If the patient has a learning disability, then the risk is increased because these youngsters typically exhibit very poor judgment. Even if the gesture or threat is in the manipulative category (see below), the youngster's poor judgment may result in the gesture's becoming an actuality. Youngsters with extremely high academic standards may become suicidal when they do not live up to their and their parents' aspirations. Disappointingly low scores on important examinations (such as the SATs) or failure to gain admission to one's first-choice college may result in suicidal attempts by such youngsters. Generally, the inordinately high standards are not simply self-imposed; most often inordinate pressures are being placed upon the youngster by parents who are obsessed with high grades and prestigious academic institutions. Impaired functioning in school, over a long period, as well as impairments in socialization increase the suicidal risk. The manipulators are more likely to be functioning adequately in these areas.

It is important for the therapist to get a good idea about the degree of stability versus instability that exists (and existed) in the adolescent's home. This cannot be done adequately without interviewing the parents, individually and jointly. Furthermore, family interviews can also be helpful in this regard. The more unhealthy and/or chaotic the youngster's home life, the greater the likelihood the suicidal gesture is genuine. Children who have been exposed to ongoing physical, psychological, and sexual abuse are much more likely to kill themselves than those who come from homes that are reasonably stable. Children from unstable homes are more likely to be runaways and suicide is more likely to occur among runaways. Obviously, a suicidal attempt made by a runaway, when away from home, is not as likely to be detected by potential rescuers and interveners. Even though the youngster may be living at home at the time of the attempt, a history of running away increases the suicidal risk. And if the parents supported the youngster's leaving the home, then the suicidal risk is also enhanced because of the parental rejection signified by such support. These are cases in which the youngsters claim that no one will care if they evaporate from the face of the earth and this may be right.

It is important to get details about the setting in which the suicidal gesture took place and the exact nature of the gesture. Youngsters who make suicidal gestures when alone are more likely to go through with it than those who do so in situations when a parent, sibling, or friend is either in the next room or expected quite soon. In the latter situation, people are being set up to "discover" the gesture before anything serious occurs. The seriousness of the gesture can also provide useful information about the youngster's true intent. If the youngster takes only a few from a large number of pills in a single bottle, then it is most unlikely that the suicidal gesture was genuine. Taking pills, even in large quantities, generally speaks for a lower level of seriousness because of the youngster's recognition of the possibility that he or she may be saved. Wrist slashing, especially when superficial, is rarely a manifestation of a bona fide suicidal attempt. If the attempt involved the use of a gun, then the risk of bona fide suicide is enhanced significantly. In fact, shooting is the most common method of committing suicide among teenagers (K. Simmons, 1987b). But even if the youngster has not threatened to use a gun, if a gun is in the home it should be removed immediately as should any pills that might be used for suicidal purposes. Hanging is also a common method used by those who are successful. Neck slashing is a very serious sign and is not only indicative of a bona fide attempt but is also strongly suggestive of the presence of psychosis. However, psychotics represent only a very small fraction of all those adolescents who successfully kill themselves. Similarly, jumping out of a window, jumping off a roof, or leaping from a high place is obviously genuine and even those who put themselves in a position where they are ready to do so are likely to be serious. However, merely threatening hysterically to take such an action—without any evidence that the youngster is inclined to do so—generally speaks for manipulation.

It is also important to investigate into the history of substance abuse. The abuse of alcohol adds to the suicidal risk. Under its influence the youngster is more likely to exhibit poor judgment and this may turn a fabricated, manipulative suicidal gesture into an actual suicide. A similar situation holds for those who abuse drugs. I am not referring here to death by overdose; I am referring here to the effect of drugs on judgment and cognition. Youngsters involved in criminal behavior are at higher risk. They may be living in dread of being prosecuted and even jailed for their criminal actions. Or, they may live in dread of retaliation for the failure to have fulfilled obligations with their criminal cohorts. I once saw in counseling the parents of a youngster who had committed suicide. The boy, himself, had never been a patient of mine. He had involved himself in both drugs and gambling and had accumulated significant debts. His criminal creditors were constantly harrassing him. In order to mollify them he would borrow more money, gamble more, and thus sunk even deeper into debt. He finally killed himself. It was clear that an important contributing factor to his suicide was the desire to bring about a cessation of his torment. Youngsters who have had difficulties with the law are often impulsive. They think primarily of the moment and do not consider enough the future consequences of their behavior. The same inpulsivity that may result in their involving themselves in criminal acts may result in their making suicidal attempts. Accordingly, the examiner does well to investigate this area, not only with regard to criminal behavior but impulsivity in other areas as well.

One should also investigate the past history of suicidal attempts. Again, one wants to get details about these—especially regarding the situations in which they occurred and the exact nature of the gestures. The greater the number of such gestures, and the more serious each of them was, the greater the likelihood that the one under consideration is serious. A past history of self-destructive behavior and accident proneness also increases the suicidal risk. It is also important to investigate into the family history of suicide. If the youngster's mother or father has indeed committed suicide, then the risk that the youngster will do so as well is significantly increased. This not only relates to the modeling element but to the privation that the youngster must have suffered following the death of the parent. This too is an extremely important differentiating criterion between the bona fide and the fabricated suicidal attempt.

Often the suicidal gesture occurs following a loss or a rejection. Accordingly, one wants to find out about previous reactions to loss or rejection, whether they were tolerated well or whether the youngster reacted severely to them. The more pathological and/or exaggerated the past reactions to loss or rejection, the greater the suicidal risk with regard to the present episode. For example, a youngster might make a suicidal gesture following rejection by a girl friend. If there has been a longstanding history of depression and exaggerated reactions to such rejections, then the likelihood that this rejection will be accompanied by a bona fide suicidal gesture is increased.

Another factor that must be considered is that of the suicide of other adolescents in the community. If the youngster's suicidal attempt was made at a time when other adolescents had committed suicide, especially others in the same area, the likelihood is increased that the youngster's attempt was genuine. This is sometimes referred to as the *cohort effect* or *copycat suicide*. Suicidal attempts, especially adolescent suicidal attempts, sometimes become epidemic. Adolescents are ever concerned with what their peers are doing and reflexively tend to go along with the "in" patterns of behavior—their professions of independence notwithstanding. One good example of this is the anorexia/bulimia phenomenon. When I was in residency training in the late 1950s, this was a relatively rare condition. At the present time anorexia/bulemia is epidemic. Articles on the subject appear consistently in teen magazines. Every classroom has at least a few such girls. And every college dorm also has its share of girls who suffer with the disorder. Suicidal attempts are no exception to the phenomenon of acquiring the psychiatric disorder in vogue at the time.

One factor that has contributed to the spread of the teen suicide phenomenon is the sensationalistic reporting of these deaths in the newspapers. This presents society with a dilemma. On the one hand, we live in a country where we pride ourselves upon our freedom of the press; to suppress, in any way, the freedom of newspapers to report such suicides would be unconstitutional. On the other hand, there is no question that the attention that such suicides provide these youngsters plays a role in encouraging others to perform similar acts. The freedom to describe them in the media, then, contributes to the death of many youngsters every year. I believe that one solution to this dilemma is for newspapers to *voluntarily* restrict such reporting to inconspicuous sections of the newspaper rather than the headlines. In this way their freedom of the press is in no way compromised and the sensationalistic contributing factor to adolescent suicide will be obviated. I recognize, however, that many newspapers will not voluntarily subscribe to this principle because it will involve a loss of income. This is just one example of the prevailing immorality and psychopathy that I see in our society.

One could ask the question here: "Okay, so the youngster is encouraged to commit suicide by the notoriety that peers have 'enjoyed' by their suicides. But don't these kids realize that suicide is final and that they won't be around to read the newspapers?" It may come as a surprise to the reader, but my answer is that they do not appreciate that they won't be around. As mentioned early in this book, one does best to view adolescents as having the bodies of adults but the brains of children. I believe that if one had the opportunity to question adolescents who kill themselves in situations in which suicide is epidemic in their communities, the vast majority would speak of some fantasy relating to their ability to appreciate and even enjoy notoriety after they have died. The fantasy involves people reading about their deaths in the newspapers, crying bitterly at their funerals, and otherwise flagellating themselves for the terrible ways in which they treated the youngster. The fantasy might include the youngster's then getting the love that is not provided in life. The fantasy might involve the youngster's being in heaven and living without the pain and the privations suffered on earth. Or the fantasy might include a degree of attention far beyond what the youngster ever enjoyed in life. And this is especially attractive to withdrawn, alienated youngsters who were ignored and/or rejected to a significant degree. Suddenly, they will be famous. The hitch, of course, is that they will not be there to enjoy their notoriety. But they somehow lose sight of this obvious fact or delude themselves into believing that it will not be that way. Some even have the fantasy that Hollywood will make a film of their lives and this, of course, will result in their becoming famous. The fantasy that they will be there to enjoy their popularity is an extension of the adolescent's delusions of invulnerability. It is also a manifestation of their cognitive simplicity.

Accordingly, therapists do well when evaluating adolescents with suicide potential to focus on this particular area. Attention to this factor has important therapeutic implications. If the youngster does indeed harbor such delusions, then the therapist should do everything to get the youngster to consider other options, options that do not include the existence of some kind of an observing spirit following death. Of course, no examiner can say with 100 percent certainty whether or not such an afterlife exists. The therapist should, however, be reasonable enough on the subject to consider the possibility that there is no such existence and to get the youngster to consider that possibility as well. But, as mentioned, even if the therapist and patient both have deep convictions for the existence of an afterlife, it is hoped that the therapist will at least take the position that the decision regarding *when* an individual should enter into that realm should not be left to an adolescent but to whatever higher forces may be involved in making it.

Another factor that should be taken into consideration when assessing the severity of the suicidal risk is the location in which the youngster lives. Most studies indicate that the rate of suicide is greater in rural areas than in the more populated urban areas. Somehow, areas with very low population density produce more suicides than those in more crowded areas. States like Nevada, Alaska, and Wyoming have suicidal rates among the highest in the country. Perhaps this relates to the isolation of such regions and the boredom that individuals living there may suffer—the beauty of their area notwithstanding. Perhaps the high rate is related to the high American Indian population in these states. This is a group that has a high suicidal rate. And this brings us to the therapist's considering the cultural factors that may be operative. In the American Indian population there is a high rate of alcoholism, unemployment, inadequate education, and a prevailing sense of hopelessness. All of these factors contribute to the higher suicidal rate in this group. But this is just one example. The therapist does well to consider the patient's socioeconomic and/or ethnic group and to investigate the suicidal rate of that group. Obviously, if it is high, then the likelihood of the patient's being suicidal is increased.

If the youngster has left a suicide note, it may be an important source of information about whether or not the attempt has been genuine. One should examine it carefully, read every word, and try to determine which of the criteria provided here are present. I am referring not only to those criteria that support bona fide attempts but fabricated attempts as well. If the note describes in detail the individuals to whom the youngster's possessions should be given, this increases the likelihood that the attempt is genuine. A suicide note in the form of a "last will and testament" also suggests serious intent. The circumstances around which the note was left and read may also provide useful information. A note mailed just before the attempt—a note that could not possibly reach the parents until *after* the death of the youngster—is more likely to be related to a serious gesture. This is also the case for unmailed notes that are not likely to be found until after death. In contrast, notes that provide advance clues to a forthcoming suicidal attempt bespeak for manipulation because they give the finders warning as well as time to interrupt the act.

Fabricated Suicidal Attempts

Now to fabricated suicidal threats and gestures. Often there is an obvious manipulative factor operating. As mentioned, such threats or gestures commonly occur in a situation in which others are present or there is every good reason to believe that others will arrive on the scene quite soon after the gesture. The motive here is to evoke guilt and to manipulate individuals into complying with certain demands. The nature of the gesture is also a telltale sign as to how serious it is. The most common fabricated gestures are wrist slashing and the ingestion of a small fraction of a bottle of pills— often pills that the youngster knows or suspects are nontoxic. In these situations one investigates into the events that led up to the suicidal gesture. Most often one will learn that the youngster has been thwarted with regard to some demand, and the gesture is an obvious attempt to get the parents to change their minds or to feel guilty over the way they have deprived the patient.

Sometimes these gestures serve to get the parents to bring the child to a therapist. Generally, this occurs in situations where the parents have refused to recognize that the youngster has problems and the suicidal attempt can thereby be viewed as a "ticket of admission into treatment." According to J.M. Toolan (1974), manipulative suicidal gestures are much more common in adolescent girls than they are in boys. My own experience bears this out. However, the sex ratio of successful attempts is just the reverse with boys successfully killing themselves much more frequently than girls. In the literature the general figures in both of these categories are four to one, i.e., four girls make attempts to every one boy who makes an attempt, but four boys are successful to every girl who is successful. Accordingly, the examiner should keep these figures in mind when making an evaluation. In short: if the patient is a girl, it is more likely that the gesture is fabricated; if the patient is a boy, it adds to the risk that the attempt is genuine (S. Wensley, 1987).

Dealing with the
Suicidal Patient's Family

I believe that if the therapist carefully considers all of the factors presented above, he or she will be in a good position to make a decision regarding whether or not the suicidal threat is genuine. However, as mentioned, in cases in which the therapist is uncertain it is best to err on the side of caution and to recommend hospitalization. If the therapist does indeed believe that the suicidal risk is present, then he or she does well to pursue one of the following courses. If the therapist believes that the risk is present, but might be reduced by intensive psychotherapy (for example three to five times a week, with the youngster and family)—and if the family is willing to become involved in such intensive treatment—then the therapist might well embark upon such a program and try to do everything possible to avoid hospitalization. But what about situations in which the family refuses both the intensive treatment program and hospitalization. In such cases I will generally remove myself from the case and send a certified letter to the family indicating that I believe that the choice is either intensive outpatient treatment or inpatient therapy. I will then state to the family that because they have refused intensive outpatient treatment and have refused hospitalization, I am discharging myself from the case and am no longer assuming any responsibility for what happens thereafter. I will be sure to include in the letter the name(s) of the hospital(s) that I would recommend they take the patient to and offer to provide recommendations for other therapists if they wish to choose the intensive outpatient treatment option with someone else.

Let us take the situation in which the therapist believes that the suicidal threat is so strong that immediate hospitalization is warranted and that the aforementioned "crash program" would be very risky. And let us consider the situation in which the patient and family refuse to go along with the recommendation for immediate hospitalization. Under these circumstances I would again write a letter in which I remove myself from the case and explain the reasons why. Again, I would strongly urge them to reconsider their decision. It is important for the reader to appreciate that such letters are written not simply because they are good psychiatry but also, considering the risks of malpractice suits at the present time, they are judicious.

Let us now consider the situation in which the family refuses hospitalization but offers the alternative of 24-hour vigils by the parents and other family members. Therapists who agree to this program should hand in their certificates. There is no justification for going along with such a reckless course. Even paid hospital attendants in an institutional setting are not consistently alert enough during their vigils to prevent hospitalized patients from suiciding on occasion. How then can one expect family members to do so? To believe that family members are going to conduct all-night vigils in rotation with one another is foolhardy and absurd. It just won't happen. Perhaps they may last a day or two, or even three, but not much longer. They are bound to slip up and they are bound to be duped by the patient who is determined to commit suicide. Accordingly, if there is indeed a bona fide suicidal risk the patient is likely to commit suicide under these circumstances. I rarely use the words *always* and *never*. However, this is one situation in which I say that the therapist should *never* be party to such an arrangement. Under these circumstances the most judicious thing for the therapist to do is to remove him- or herself from the case with an associated letter of explanation. In it, of course, the therapist must advise the parents to seek hospitalization.

MEDICATION

Introduction

I am in full agreement with those who claim that "for every crooked thought there must be a crooked molecule." There must be a neurological basis for all symptoms. There are some, however, who claim that this dictum makes the differentiation between the psychogenic and organic an anachronism, a residuum of medieval thinking. They would consider such differentiations to be in the category of questions like how many angels can dance on the head of a pin. Although I believe that it is true that there must be a neurological basis for all thoughts and feelings—because one must have a nerve cell to have a thought or a feeling—I do not believe that it necessarily follows that the differentiation between psychogenic and organic symptoms is irrelevant in these modern times. Such differentiation concerns itself with the crucial question of *how* the molecule got "crooked." This is important because the more we know about the pathogenesis of a disorder, the better the likelihood we will be able to do something about it.

In addition, the differentiation has important therapeutic implications. If one believes that the molecule got crooked because of environmental (especially family) influences, then one is more likely to recommend psychotherapy, milieu therapy, family therapy, and other therapeutic approaches that involve personality changes in the patient and his or her associates. In contrast, if one believes that the etiology is metabolic, genetic, biological, etc. then one is more likely to have little faith in the therapeutic efficacy of environmental changes and more conviction that some drug (presently or in the future) will straighten out the molecule. This may very well be the case. This does not, however, negate the aforementioned arguments. Knowledge is power and the more we know about the etiology of a disorder the better we will be able to prevent and treat it. In addition, most of those who use medication in psychiatry will agree that they do not provide complete cures, that whatever straightening of the molecules such drugs can achieve, they still remain somewhat twisted. Accordingly, at this present state of our knowledge (or more accurately ignorance) we do well to utilize all therapeutic modalities, both biological and environmental.

Antidepressants

Compared to other psychiatrists, I consider myself to have a somewhat conservative position on prescribing medication. With regard to medication for depression, I recognize that my position is a rare one in psychiatry today, because I consider the vast majority of depressions to be psychogenic in etiology. With the exception of people with manic-depressive psychosis (still rare in my opinion), the overwhelming majority of people I see who are depressed are so because of psychogenic factors. This does not preclude the presence of a genetic predisposition. Nor does my position preclude the belief that depressed patients can be helped by antidepressant medication. It is probably the case that the antidepressant does not differentiate between depressions that are biological in etiology and those that are environmentally or psychologically induced. However, I believe that the psychiatrist who confines him- or herself to antidepressant medication only, is not dealing with many if not most of the fundamental problems that have contributed to the development of the patient's depression. Although one may achieve with medication some symptomatic alleviation of the depression, one should still be dealing with the life situations that have contributed to its formation and perpetuation.

Viewing depression as primarily, if not exclusively, biological in etiology is attractive because it enables the therapist to prescribe medication only and not involve him- or herself in the more arduous and expensive task of ongoing psychotherapy for the patient and possibly family members. Viewing depression to be primarily if not exclusively biological in etiology is "cost effective," enables therapists to "treat" large numbers of people, and is attractive to hospital administrators, agencies, and those who fund treatment. Rather than view the vast majority of depressed people as being the unfortunate victims of a metabolic disease, I generally approach the problem with the question: "What is the person depressed about?" I believe that depression is being overly diagnosed because making the diagnosis provides the therapist with justification for prescribing antidepressant medication—a quick and easy cure. In recent years, we are told by newspapers, magazines, and psychiatrists that depression is much more common than people previously realized, but there is no reason to lose heart because we have recently enjoyed "good news about depression" and the good news is that doctors have now discovered "miracle" cures. Magazine articles abound describing people who were treated unsuccessfully by psychotherapy for many years and then quickly cured in one or two sessions by a biological psychiatrist. Individual testimonies generally are considered proof that the antidepressant produced the "cure." My own view is that in the last 15 or 20 years, there has been "bad news about depression" in that the emphasis on the biological etiology has diverted people from focusing on its psychodynamics. And this, I believe, is really bad news for people who are depressed. It is also bad news for psychiatry.

Thus far, I have not seen fit to prescribe antidepressant medication for children. Nor have I prescribed it for younger adolescents. On those rare occasions when I have prescribed it for youngsters in the mid- to late-adolescent period, I have found the serotonin reuptake inhibitors to be the most efficacious. But, even when I do prescribe medication, I combine it with intensive psychotherapy. And I make it known to the patient and family that I view antidepressant medication to be an *adjunct* to the primary treatment, which is psychotherapy and the working out of the complex personal and family problems that have contributed to the development and perpetuation of the patient's symptoms.

Lithium

When I attended medical school in the mid-1950s we were taught that the manic-depressive psychosis is an extremely rare disorder and we considered ourselves fortunate in being able to see such a patient demonstrated to one of our classes. In the late 1950s lithium was introduced as one of the most predictable and effective treatments for the manic phase of manic-depressive psychosis. As the years rolled on, more and more people became diagnosed as having manic-depressive psychosis and various other kinds of manic disorders. I do not believe that there has been any increase in the actual incidence or prevalence of this disorder. What has increased is the frequency with which psychiatrists have diagnosed it, in order to justify giving such patients lithium. So enthusiastic have psychiatrists been about prescribing lithium that it is often even given for people who are depressed, under the theory that it will "flatten" the bipolar fluctuations. And an ever-expanding list of people have been diagnosed as having manic episodes: people who are agitated, hyperactive adolescents (and even preadolescents), anxious people, those who speak under tension, people who go on spending splurges (even though not psychotic), individuals who talk too quickly, and anyone else for whom the psychiatrist wishes to justify prescribing lithium.

I do believe that lithium does help reduce mania in patients suffering with bona fide manic states. I do *not* believe that it alleviates depression and I do *not* believe that it helps people who are *not* genuinely manic. Again, we see a situation in which a good drug is overutilized by psychiatrists who diagnose everyone and anyone who might have symptoms that might justify the drug's utilization. Such overdiagnosing lessens our sense of therapeutic impotence and creates in us the delusion that we can cure more people than we actually can. In the service of this goal bipolar disorders are then suddenly discovered to be more prevalent than previously realized. Armies of new experts now crop up in the service of the same needs. Expert diagnosticians then claim that they have seen incipient manic behavior, early phases of manic behavior, etc., all in the service of justifying prescribing lithium. Here too, investigation into the psychodynamics of the excited states need not be done, all one needs do is prescribe lithium— which is far more efficient, quick, and "cost effective."

Neuroleptics
and Anxiolytics

Although I recognize the value of phenothiazines and other neuroleptics in the treatment of psychotic states, I have had little opportunity to use them in recent years because of my limited experience with psychotic children. I have had more experience with anxiolytic agents, especially diazepam (Valium). I have used diazepam in the treatment of children with separation anxiety disorder and consider it to be of some symptomatic value. However, the primary focus of my treatment of such children is on the symbiotic relationship they most often have with their mothers and on the other psychogenic problems that these children have. R. Gittelman-Klein, and D.F. Klein (1973) and R. Gittelman-Klein (1975) consider imipramine (Tofranil), a tricyclic antidepressant, to be useful in the treatment of separation anxiety disorder. They believe that it blocks the peripheral manifestations of the panic state. Although my experience with imipramine for this purpose has been limited, I have not found it significantly useful in the treatment of these children. One difficulty in assessing its efficacy in the treatment of panic states is that it generally takes a week or two before its effect can be assessed. Diazepam, in contrast, generally works within a half hour and I believe is much more likely to reduce anxiety and panic. I have also prescribed diazepam for children who are severely anxious. One of the problems with diazepam is that youngsters taking it can easily become lethargic in school and so one must become quite careful in monitoring the dosage level.

Psychostimulants

I consider myself to have had extensive experience with psychostimulants, especially methylphenidate (Ritalin), dextroamphetamine (Dexadrine), and pemoline (Cylert). I consider these drugs to be useful for children with hyperactivity, but I do not consider them to be of any value in helping youngsters sustain attention. I consider it important to differentiate between hyperactivity and the impairment in sustaining attention (the so-called attention-deficit disorder). Elsewhere (1987b) I have discussed studies of mine that, I believe, clearly support my view that true attention deficit disorder (ADD) is very rare. Hyperactivity, however, certainly is to be found, but is best considered to be a manifestation of temperamental, genetically determined, high activity level. I believe that psychostimulant medications do three things: 1) reduce hyperactivity, 2) enhance compliance with parents and teachers, and 3) reduce impulsivity. When parents are asked whether psychostimulant medication has helped their youngster, a common reply is: "Doctor, he listens better when he's taking the medicine." When such parents use the words "listens better" in these situations, they are not referring to attention-sustaining capacity; rather, they are referring to the child's *compliance*. If one investigates further into whether or not hyperactive children also have ADD, one will often learn from parents that they will sit for hours watching television and generally have no problem concentrating on their favorite TV programs. I generally prefer methylphenidate and dextroamphetamine over pemoline because of the latter's time lag before becoming effective. Dextroamphetamine and methylphenidate generally work within 30 to 45 minutes, whereas pemoline does not build up to effective dosage levels until seven to ten days. Furthermore, it is much easier for me to monitor the former drugs with my Steadiness Tester (Gardner, 1979, Gardner et al., 1979), to objectively ascertain whether or not the drug is being effective in reducing hyperactivity. I can also use it to monitor the dosage levels in order to ascertain the level of optimum efficacy.

HOSPITALIZATION

Introduction

I consider myself to have a very conservative position with regard to hospitalizing adolescent patients. I do believe that there certainly are indications for hospitalizing a youngster in this age bracket, but I also believe that the majority of adolescent patients who are presently hospitalized would not have been so had I been the one to make the decision. I generally view hospitalization to be warranted primarily for people who are homicidal, suicidal, or who are in very special situations (to be described below) where it is only by separation from their families that there is any hope for alleviation of their difficulties. Most patients' problems have both intrapsychic and interpersonal contributory elements. The therapist must work in both areas. This usually involves individual work and close work with family members. Plucking the person out of the family context, putting the individual in the hospital, and then treating that person in isolation from the family in the hope that such treatment will help the individual reintegrate him- or herself into the family is often misguided. Doing everything possible to keep the patient in the family, the environment wherein the problems arose and the environment wherein the problems are best worked through is, in my opinion, the preferable approach.

The Medical Model

I believe that one factor that contributes to the ease with which many therapists hospitalize relates to the influence of the medical model on psychiatric practice. Although it is true that the hospital may very well be the optimum place for the treatment of many physical disorders, it does not necessarily follow that the hospital is also the best place for the treatment of many psychiatric disorders. The reflex hospitalization of the patient often reflects doctors' blindly following the medical model.

The Hospital Business

It is important for the reader to appreciate (if he or she doesn't already) that many hospitals are basically businesses, often run and owned by nonmedical people. This is not only the case for private hospitals but, more recently, even for nonprofit and voluntary hospitals as well. Under these circumstances an empty bed means loss of income. The criteria for hospitalization then become expanded—often to include any situation that might justify hospitalization, no matter how weak the justifications. Many fancy and well-appointed hospitals charge enormous amounts of money (hundreds of dollars a day) and are nothing more than hotels. They look good on paper with regard to the kind of staff that is providing treatment, but little meaningful therapy is provided. In such facilities one of the most important (if not the most important) determinants of how long a patient will stay will be how much money the individual has. All other criteria are of secondary importance in determining the length of hospitalization. When the person runs out of insurance coverage (inevitable with such prices), the staff is suddenly talking about discharge from the hospital. At that point the patient is referred back to the referring physician, just as a specialist in a hospital might refer back a patient to a referring general practitioner. The notion of the importance of continuity of treatment and the all-important ongoing therapist-patient relationship are of little concern to those in the hospital business. When they say that the average patient stays 21 days in their hospital, they would like to imply that that was all the patients needed and that they were significantly improved and even "cured" following their sojourn in the facility. What the 21-day average really means is that that was just about all most of their patients could possibly afford before being forcibly discharged.

It is also important for the reader to appreciate that psychiatry is also a business and that a psychiatrist referring a patient for hospitalization may do so more for financial gain than therapeutic indications. Most psychiatrists follow traditional practice in their private offices and charge a specific fee for a traditional 45 to 50 minute session. At this time (1988), the going rate for most psychiatrists is somewhere between $75 and $125 per session. In a hospital, however, one "makes rounds" (again, following the medical model). A patient may be seen for only five or ten minutes and the psychiatrist may easily get away with charging not only standard fees but even more because insurance companies tend to pay more money for people who are in hospitals. Under these circumstances earning $1000 in an hour is not uncommon. And when patients complain about this, they are told that their disgruntlement is just another manifestation of their psychopathology and that if they were healthier they wouldn't be complaining so much. (No wonder so many people hate the psychiatrists they see in such hospitals.)

The Teaching Hospital

Another factor that contaminates the decision regarding hospitalization relates to the situation in teaching hospitals, those closely affiliated with medical schools. These hospitals have an obligation to provide patients for medical students, interns, and residents. In addition, most teaching hospitals train psychologists, psychiatric social workers, and sometimes nurse practitioners, pastoral counselors, and others who want to become therapists. It would seriously compromise the reputation of such an institution if it did not have a good supply of patients for all these students and their teachers. Once again, the criteria for hospitalization become loosened in order to provide such "teaching material."

Situations in Which Hospitalization is Warranted

The Chaotic, Disorganized Home   The aforementioned contaminations regarding admission criteria notwithstanding, there are still patients who do need to be removed from their families. Occasionally, the patient's home life may be so chaotic and the family so incapable of working through their problems that the only way to prevent further deterioration of the youngster is to remove him or her from the home. Under these circumstances, the hospital may be viewed as a way station to placement elsewhere. These are situations in which the family has proven itself to be unworkable regarding any kind of therapeutic intervention. Such "crisis intervention" is certainly indicated. However, even then, day hospitals will sometimes serve (J.C. Westman, 1979). Under these circumstances the hospitals may provide a structure that does not exist in the home. The environment is far more predictable than the chaotic one of the home. And these factors are generally salutary.

It is important for therapists to appreciate that even under these circumstances, there are certain elements in the hospital program that are antitherapeutic. I have already mentioned the lack of continuity of treatment and the lack of appreciation of an ongoing therapist-relationship as the cornerstone of effective psychotherapy. Another drawback is that the youngster is being placed in an environment with other disturbed adolescents, adolescents who may be suffering with moderately severe to severe psychiatric disorders. Whatever benefit may be derived from the healthy therapeutic milieu of the administration and caretaking personnel, there is no question that exposure to other sick adolescents has many antitherapeutic elements. Certainly, one of the aims of treatment is to help the adolescent relate better to peers. But with peers who are severely disturbed, more unhealthy than healthy behavior may be learned. It is common for parents, when visiting such facilities, to comment that their youngster will be placed with a lot of "crazy kids." Traditionally, such parents are reassured that there is nothing antitherapeutic or dangerous about such placement and that their concerns are unwarranted. At best, this is naive; at worst, the reassurance is duplicitous. It is often not believed by the reassurer but he or she doesn't want to lose a "good customer."

Jacob Christ (1974) puts it well:

> Whenever possible the treatment of an adolescent problem situation should first be attempted on an outpatient basis and with active participation of the family. Even in cases where

psychotic syndromes are present, much understanding can often be gained from an exploration on an individual and family basis. Institutionalization for acute situations should be reserved for life-threatening circumstances. For chronic situations, it will be important first and foremost to assess the strength of the youngster and the family's resources to deal with a given problem. Repetitive crises, which often occur in the matrix of a chronic unsatisfactory situation, can sometimes be dealt with by crisis intervention methods. However, where it has become clear that neither the teenager nor the family has means at their disposal to extricate themselves from a destructive situation, a change in milieu may be necessary. It is in those circumstances that school away from home or institutionalization may be necessary. A structured milieu often has beneficial effects in those cases where clearly no structure had been provided by the parents and where either physical or emotional deprivation had been a problem. It needs to be understood that institutionalization for chronic problems will usually require some considerable time, and the adolescent hospitalized or institutionalized will often fight hard battles with the caring personnel.

Christ mentions that the patients "will often fight hard battles with caring personnel." These battles are often viewed as manifestations of the patient's psychopathology. Unfortunately, this is often not the case. Some of the sickest people gravitate toward jobs in psychiatric hospitals. Many are borderline and some even psychotic. Many are sadistic, psychopathic, or just plain lazy and uninterested. Accordingly, I would rephrase Christ's statement: "will often fight hard battles with *uncaring* personnel." This is another reason for therapists' thinking twice before recommending hospitalization, even for those from chaotic, unstructured homes.

Antisocial Acting Out   Elsewhere in this book (especially in Chapter One) I discussed the treatment of antisocial disorders in some detail. Here I focus on certain aspects of the treatment of such youngsters related to the issue of hospitalization. Office and clinic treatment is for patients who do not pose a threat to the therapist's person or property. If the therapist has to work under circumstances in which he or she fears harm to him- or herself or destruction of his or her property, then effective psychotherapy is not likely to be possible. The enhanced attention and vigilance associated with such concerns of being harmed by the patient cannot but compromise the therapist's objectivity. Patients who threaten such damage should be told that outpatient treatment is for those who *talk* about their problems rather than those who *act out* on them, especially against their therapists. Although not all patients who threaten harm to their therapists and/or act out against them should necessarily be sent to a hospital, most of them are not reasonably considered candidates for psychotherapy. The alternatives for such patients, then, are either no treatment at all or treatment in a hospital setting where the therapist can be comforted by the protection (not always perfect, to say the least) of the hospital staff. With less tension and vigilance on the therapist's part, there is a greater likelihood that he or she can attend to the patient's problems.

Hospitalization must seriously be considered for antisocial youngsters whose behavior is so dangerous that there is a real risk of homicide. On occasion this relates to reckless driving when inebriated or under the influence of drugs. On other occasions the patient is engaging in such violent antisocial acts that there is a real danger that someone will be killed.

Behavior Modification as a Treatment for Antisocial Adolescents   Most hospitals for adolescents provide behavior modification programs. These have been very much in vogue during the last 15 to 20 years and are certainly considered far more "cost effective" than something as inefficient as long-term psychotherapy. I believe that behavior modification programs—as the primary, if not exclusive, modality for antisocial acting out—do more harm than good. I wish to emphasize that I am confining myself here to the use of behavior modification in the treatment of *antisocial disorders*, and I am *not* commenting on the use of behavior modification for the treatment of other disorders such as phobias, for example.

To elaborate. Although behavior therapists differ with regard to their conviction for the role in which underlying psychodynamics contribute to symptom formation, when they use behavior modification therapeutically, they are focusing primarily, if not exclusively, on symptomatic alleviation or removal. For many the symptoms *are* essentially the disease. But even those who have some conviction for the importance of psychodynamic factors in bringing about symptoms, the focus is on symptom removal when behavior modification is utilized. Generally, this is done by providing *positive reinforcement* for desirable behavior. An example of this would be praise or, more formally, rewarding the child with tokens, candy, merit points, or some other desirable item. In addition, attempts to discourage the child from undesirable behavior are made by utilizing *negative reinforcement*. Here, an aversive stimulus that has been applied to discourage the perpetuation and repetition of the behavior is removed. An example of this would be the cessation of scolding a child after he or she has exhibited undesirable behavior or lifting a restriction that has been imposed after exhibiting undesirable behavior. Another technique utilized in behavior modification is *punishment*. Here, an aversive stimulus is applied following undesirable behavior in an attempt to suppress that behavior in the future. An example of this would be placing the child in a locked room, often given a euphemistic name such as "quiet room." Last, *extinction* is also used. Here, an attempt is made to discourage undesirable behavior by suppressing factors that reinforce it. An example of this would be ignoring a youngster who has a tantrum or rage outburst rather than paying attention to him or her. Further details on these approaches are described by I.G. Sarason and B.R. Sarason (1980).

I view these approaches to be, at best, superficial. But when applied as the primary, if not exclusive, mode of treatment for antisocial behavior, they are not only destructive but perpetuate the very symptoms that they are designed to discourage or "extinguish." The latter term is extremely misleading because the approach is just the opposite. They actually entrench the very behavior that they are designed to obliterate. The entrenchment does not take place at the time of the application of the aversive stimuli and negative reinforcement. Rather, it takes place after the youngster is out of the hospital, after the therapists have written their articles describing the wonderful results they have obtained with behavior modification.

To elaborate on this point. Youngsters with antisocial behavior disorders, as described in detail in Vol. I (1999a), have defects in the development of the internal guilt-evoking mechanisms (conscience). The therapeutic approach *must* attempt to strengthen these youngsters' sense of guilt. I use the word guilt here, as I have previously, to refer to the feeling of lowered self-worth that the individual experiences after having thoughts, experienced feelings, or committed acts that the person has learned in childhood are wrong or bad. These youngsters need *more* guilt and the therapist should do everything possible to make them feel more guilty. Behavior modification misses this important point. The alleged guilt that a graduate of these behavior modification programs feels, if anything, is more like the guilt that the judge is referring to when he asks an accused whether or not he pleads guilty or innocent. Here, the judge is basically asking whether the individual admits to having committed the crime or not. Nothing is said about intrapsychic processes that may or may not be operative. Actually, we should have two different words to refer to these phenomena—so apart are they. Behavior modification teaches youngsters to deter themselves from performing unacceptable acts by the awareness that if they do so, they will suffer some kind of pain or some pleasure will be removed. Nothing is likely to be said about the victim and no attempt is generally made to internalize the inhibitory mechanisms. Behavior modification deals with externals. Psychotherapy focuses on internals, yet it need not ignore externals (as I have demonstrated so often throughout this book).

Behavior modification is less likely to devote itself to the more formidable task of investigation into intrapsychic processes because it is not "cost effective" and is a far more demanding and time-consuming task. In a behavior modification program, when a youngster is anticipating an antisocial act, he calculates the risk of being caught and what the consequences will be. In a "good" behavior modification program he is able to predict with a fair degree of accuracy exactly what is going to happen to him if caught. He may or may not decide to take his chances. But, even if he does commit the transgression and is caught, he can often "work off" the demerits, punishments, etc. by good works. Accordingly, the system teaches various kinds of manipulations.

Once these youngsters have been "cured" and discharged from the hospital they find themselves in a world completely unlike that of the hospital. No one is walking around with clipboards and check lists. No one is giving them merits and demerits, rewards and punishments, and putting these into a computer. Without such monitoring, and without their having developed any internalized inhibitory mechanisms, they bounce back and become even worse than they were before. It is then that I see them in my office. When I have made these criticisms to people who work in such programs, I am sometimes told that individual psychotherapy is also provided and that attempts are made to instill guilt as well. Although I cannot say that this never takes place, I am somewhat dubious that it is the prevailing approach. First, in most of these facilities, there is not the time to provide intensive individual therapy to all of the patients. Next, the staff personnel are generally not schooled in intensive psychotherapy, rather they are committed more to the seemingly easier and ostensibly more efficient behavior modification.

Other Situations for Which Hospitalization May Be Warranted   I have already mentioned bona fide suicidal gestures as a justifiable and even compelling reason for hospitalization. Some adolescent youngsters may need hospitalization for the treatment of drug abuse, because they cannot be trusted to wean themselves from the habit in a noncontrolled situation. Girls suffering with bulimia/anorexia may require hospitalization. These patients generally require a hospital setting in which the personnel are particularly familiar with the treatment of such youngsters. Otherwise, they tend to manipulate hospital personnel into the same kinds of pathological transactions and "games" that they have involved themselves in with their parents. Starving themselves is not unknown among such patients and the likelihood that this can take place may be reduced by removing the youngster from the family milieu in which the symptom is thriving. Because some of these patients literally starve themselves to death, hospitalization in such cases may be lifesaving.

CONCLUDING COMMENTS

I recognize that some readers may consider me to have a somewhat jaundiced view of the value of hospitalization for adolescent patients. It is a view derived primarily from the "outside." What I have seen of the "inside" comes from my residency days as well as my experiences over 25 years as an attending psychiatrist at the New York State Psychiatric Institute at the Columbia-Presbyterian Medical Center. There I have supervised residents who have patients admitted to the inpatient service. My experience has been that the younger the patient the less the likelihood I would have recommended hospitalization. This is certainly the case for many, if not most, on the children's inpatient service. With regard to adolescents, the same principle holds. My experience has been that the younger adolescents, generally, are less likely to require hospitalization than some of the older ones. And the older ones have generally been youngsters with flagrant psychotic episodes which, I will agree, probably do require hospitalization because of the danger to themselves and others if they are not placed in a protected setting. The reader who is interested in further discussion of the subject of hospitalization of adolescent patients does well to refer to articles by D.B. Rinsley (1974), L.A. Stone (1979), and D. Zinn (1979).

THREE

CONCLUDING COMMENTS AND A LOOK AT THE FUTURE

Although the primary purpose of this book has been to focus on specific psychotherapeutic techniques of use in the treatment of adolescents, I have throughout commented on family and environmental changes that might be therapeutically beneficial for them. I have not, however, discussed in detail how the therapist might bring about changes in the environment. Rather, I have focused my attention primarily on the psychotherapeutic techniques that the therapist might utilize in his or her office when working directly with the patient. Therapists who choose to involve themselves in bringing about these broader changes in society are contributing to the advancement of preventive psychiatry. Obviously, a single individual is only capable of making a small contribution in this realm. However, the greater the number of therapists who involve themselves beyond their offices in bringing about these changes, the greater the likelihood they will come about.

Therapists like myself who devote themselves primarily to individual psychotherapy generally have little time left over for extensive involvement in such causes. However, this does not preclude some involvement. And if these small degrees of involvement are multiplied by large numbers of therapists, then an impact may be made. Therapists do well to think intermittently about these issues and, in the course of their daily living, take those opportunities that may come their way to promulgate their particular causes. Public speaking and writing provide excellent vehicles for spreading one's ideas and therapists do well to avail themselves of such opportunities when they arise. Volumes could be written on the various kinds of social changes that might be psychologically useful for adolescents, both at the preventive and therapeutic levels. Here I will focus on a few areas that are of particular concern to me. Some of these points have already been made in the course of the book, but I repeat them here because I believe they are worthy of emphasis and reiteration.

CHILD CARE

First, I would like to emphasize that I am in sympathy with and support of the feminist movement. There is no question that women have been subjected to terrible persecution and other indignities throughout the course of history and there is no question that we have a long way to go until we reach the point of full egalitarianism. Also, I wish to emphasize at the outset that I am in full support of women being given the opportunity to pursue and work within any career, occupation, or skill. However, just about every social advance is associated with untoward reactions, drawbacks, and undesirable effects—many of which are unforeseen. And women's entrance into the extradomestic realm is no exception to this phenomenon. I focus here on the effects of such liberation on children. Whatever benefits may be derived by women as a result of their changing roles from child rearer to bread winner, there is no question that many children have suffered. The simple facts are that to the degree that the mother invests herself in professional fulfillment she is neglecting her children. But this is true of fathers as well. And I am not referring here simply to the effects of the time parents spend out of the home, but their psychological investment in the extra-domestic activities. When one comes home at the end of the day drained and exhausted, there is little *quality* involvement left over for the children.

As more mothers have entered the workplace, an increasing number of children have been left to the care of others. Many are put in day-care centers and many are left with friends, relatives, and neighbors. The more remote the caretaking individuals are from the mother (biologically and psychologically) the less the likelihood these children will receive optimum care. And the younger the children, the greater the likelihood they will develop psychological problems. The simple facts are these: the biological parent is much more likely to provide optimum care than anyone else on earth. I don't care how many Ph.D.s the people at the day-care center have and I don't care how committed they are to the child-rearing process, they are still not likely to have as strong a psychological bond with the children under their care as the biological mother. And then there is the turnover. They can't possibly maintain ongoing strong ties with children who are being replaced every year or two. And even if ties are formed, they are broken by the structure of the system. This too is detrimental. In line with my theory of the development of the internalized guilt-evoking mechanisms described in Vol. I (1999a), I believe that this phenomenon is *one* of the factors operative in producing psychopathic personality types. It is *one* of the factors involved in the erosion of values and morals that I see in our society.

As mentioned earlier in this series, I believe there is a relatively simple solution to this problem. It is rare that I can make such a statement. Most problems are exceedingly complex and it is extremely unusual to be able to say that there is a simple solution. But there is one for this problem. Specifically, we can reasonably restructure our society so that both fathers and mothers alternate work outside the home two to three days a week and spend two to three days within the home during each work week. Both could be home on weekends. And this program is feasible. All of us have had the experience of calling an office and asking to speak with Mr. Jones. We are told that Jones is not available on that day but will be available on the next day; we are asked if we would like to speak with Smith. Under the system I propose here, Jones would be home with his baby rather than merely out of the office working for the company elsewhere. As children get older and attend school, parents could then expand their involvements outside the home. I am not claiming that this program could be easily implemented; I am only claiming that it is feasible and realizable. The vast majority of offices, businesses, and industries can accomodate such a work program for their employees.

Implementation of this plan would not preclude entirely the function of child-care centers. Rather, a smaller percentage of child-care could still be provided by them. I am not claiming that the child-care center experience is 100 percent detrimental to children. They do learn socialization and are provided with opportunities to expand their emotional and intellectual horizons. My main criticism is the quantity of time that many children are spending there and, in many cases, the poor quality of care provided. I believe that society would benefit immensely if the aforementioned parental work plan were implemented because healthier children would develop from it. And healthier children become healthier adults, and strengthen thereby society at large.

I believe also that elderly people are not being properly used in the child-rearing process. Many older people are still quite capable of providing meaningful child care, their infirmities notwithstanding. They often have the time and the patience to take care of children, and such involvement may provide meaning to lives that may otherwise appear meaningless. On occasion I have read or heard about child-care centers that have linked up with old-age homes, much to the benefit of both institutions. Elderly people could also be involved significantly in the operation of child-care centers. I understand that in China this is routinely done. Specifically, while both parents are working out in the fields or in the factories, elderly people take care of the children. They assist in the care of pre-schoolers in day-care centers and involve themselves, as well, in after-school care for older children.

THE PSYCHOLOGICAL PROBLEMS
OF BLACK CHILDREN

It is now almost 125 years since the end of the Civil War. Everyone agrees that things have not changed significantly for black children.

Since that time waves of immigrants from practically every country in the world have come to these shores, and each group has somehow found its path into the mainstream of middle America. Except the blacks. Recently, I heard a series of speakers commenting on the fact that now, twenty years after the death of Martin Luther King, very little has changed for the vast majority of black people. All agreed the problems are complex and just about all claimed that one of the things that was needed was more money. Some mentioned that some of the more recent immigrants—especially Chinese, Japanese, Koreans, Indians, and Vietnamese—are moving rapidly into the mainstream of American life and their children are receiving a wide variety of prestigious academic awards. The explanation given for this disparity is the inferior education black children receive in inner cities. I do not question that this is a factor. However, not one speaker spoke about what I consider to be a primary element in explaining the failure of blacks to move ahead into the mainstream of American society.

The basic problem of black children is the absence of a father figure in the home from birth through the formative years. The primary adult model for millions of black children is the mother figure only. And for millions this mother may be a teenager who is still a child being taken care of by her own mother, the infant's maternal grandmother. The child's father is often unknown, or if known is often only intermittently involved, or not involved at all in the child-rearing process. There are few, if any, male models for educational aspiration and/or the extra-domestic work ethic. But there may be models for psychopathic behavior provided by males in the streets who are often involved significantly in crime and drugs. As cited previously in this book, a number of years ago one of the black comedians—I think it was Dick Gregory—made comments along these lines to a group of blacks: "You want to be successful in life? I'll tell you how to be successful in life. Get up in the morning, take a pencil and paper, follow an Oriental around all day, and write down exactly what he does. Then, starting the next day, you do exactly the same things." I don't care how much money is spent in helping blacks. It is not likely to work if some of the money is not spent in the realm of educating people to this important fact. All the other groups who have entered into America's mainstream have had strong family ties in which parents were involved with children throughout the full course of their upbringing. When I say parents I mean both mothers and fathers, each playing his or her own role in the child-rearing process. It would be an error for the reader to conclude that I am proposing this as the entire solution to the problem of blacks in America. Rather, I am stating that it is a special problem which, if not solved, will make all other efforts futile. It may be difficult to bring about changes in this pattern in a short time. It will probably take many generations. However, without drawing attention to the problem, the first steps toward its alleviation are not likely to be taken.

DIVORCE AND CUSTODY LITIGATION

Another common source of psychopathology in children that could be avoided is that which is associated with divorce and custody litigation. I am not referring here to the psychopathology that may arise directly as a result of the divorce; rather, I am referring to the unnecessary and additional psychopathology that results from the exposure of children to and their embroilment in their parents' divorce and custody litigation. People who are divorcing have enough grief; they don't need the additional stress associated with having to litigate. In most countries of the world people do not have to litigate in order to get a divorce. In the United States, probably more than anywhere else in the world, people who are divorcing become subjected to the additional psychological traumas of adversary litigation. However, for most people in the U.S. there is an option that is not being utilized widely enough. I am referring to mediation. There is no reason why the vast majority of people who divorce should not go first to a mediator who will help them resolve their differences. In order to ensure that the final agreement is truly impartial, each of the parents could have the document reviewed by his or her own attorney who would assess the instrument for inequities. These independent attorneys should be individuals who serve themselves as mediators in other cases. They should not be lawyers who are the barracuda types who relish adversary litigation with little heed to the psychological toll on their clients and with primary concern for the amount of money they can extract from them. If either party or either adversary attorney considered inequities to be present in the agreement derived from the mediation process, then the three attorneys (the mediator and the two independent counselors) could meet together to attempt to iron out any differences that may still be present. Then, the two attorneys could obtain for their clients a noncontested divorce. If the mediator felt the need for consultation with a child psychiatrist (if there were a custody conflict) or an accountant (if complex financial problems arose) then he or she could do so. If, however, the mediation breaks down and the parties are not able to resolve their differences, then they might still have the opportunity to resort to adversary litigation. Of course, there are other mediation programs, but the aforementioned is the one that I prefer.

People divorcing today are easy prey to an army of attorneys who are exploiting them. At the present time there is approximately one attorney for every 800 people in the population. Clearly, all these attorneys cannot possibly make a living as lawyers. Accordingly, there are many "hungry" attorneys, but there is a sea of gullible people who are allowing themselves to be exploited by them. About ten years ago mediation began to move forward and I had hopes that by the end of this century it would be the routine method for obtaining a divorce. Unfortunately, it appears to me that the initial momentum is dying down. From the outset lawyers resisted the movement because of the obvious fact that two lawyers engaging their clients in protracted adversary litigation will bring in far more money to the profession than one lawyer serving as a mediator. Furthermore, ours is very much an adversarial society — the most litigious country on earth (J. K. Lieberman, 1981) — and mediation goes very much against this philosophy. About eight years ago, I wrote that by the end of this century people would look back on the mid- to late-20th century as a time of national craziness with regard to the quickness with which individuals involved themselves in adversary litigation for divorce and custody disputes. I suspect that this prophecy will not be realized and the exploitation of divorcing people will continue into the 21st century as will the sadistic destruction of parents and children that is fomented by embroilment in adversary litigation. Elsewhere (1986) I have discussed in detail the wide variety of psychological disorders, both in parents and in children, that can result from protracted divorce and custody litigation.

THE AMERICAN EDUCATIONAL SYSTEM

I have mentioned in this book the drawbacks of a seemingly egalitarian educational system which assumes that "all children are created equal" and that all children should receive the same educational exposures. I consider this to be misguided egalitarianism that must blind itself to the obvious intellectual differences that children exhibit from the time of birth. On the one hand, educators appreciate that every intelligence test has its bell-shaped curve. On the other hand, the educational system does not properly accommmodate these differences. I do not claim that there is no appreciation at all of these differences; I only claim that not enough appreciation to these differences is given. Although there are special classes for learning-disabled children, and although there are technical high schools for those who are not academically inclined, the main thrust and orientation of our educational system is toward preparing youngsters to enter colleges and universities. The ideal presented to all youngsters is that they should ultimately be able to attend one of these so-called institutions of higher learning.

Most of the other countries on earth have no problem accepting the fact that not all children should be on a strong academic track. Accordingly, somewhere between the ages of 9 and 11 they are divided into three tracks. The highest track ultimately leads to the university. The lowest track ends formal heavy academic training at about age 11 or 12 and emphasizes various trades and skills. And the middle track is somewhere between the two. Of course, if the child has been placed in the wrong track, there is still a possibility of switching. We would do well in the United States to institute such a system. It would save a lot of children a lot of grief. To say that all people should be *treated* equally before the *law* is certainly reasonable. But to say that all are *created* equal is absurd. What is more reasonable to say (and I don't know who first said it) is that "some are more equal than others." Because public statements of such inegalitarianism are considered undemocratic in our society at this time, it is extremely unlikely that such changes will be introduced into our system in the foreseeable future, certainly not before the end of this century.

I have also mentioned at various points in this book the "college disease" wherein parents suffer terrible humiliation if their children do not go to college. This too is an extension of the all-men-are-created-equal principle. I believe that about 10 to 15 percent of all colleges in the United States are genuinely institutions of higher learning. The rest are merely businesses catering to a gullible population that needs to believe that it is important that children go to college. And the children comply by spending four years in these "educational" centers. They learn something about drinking, drugs, and sex; but they learn little else. Yes, they go through the formal courses, they take examinations, and they get grades. Yet the whole thing does not add up to an education. It adds up to four years of recreation and more dependency. It does not prepare most of these youngsters to function in real life. In most of these institutions it is very difficult to "flunk out." After all, a good businessman does not throw a paying customer out of the store. And grade inflation will ensure that even the feeble-minded obtain high grades, fostering thereby the delusion that something is being learned. I doubt whether this situation will change very much by the end of the century either.

THE FUTURE OF THE FIELD OF
PSYCHODYNAMIC PSYCHOTHERAPY

Unfortunately, at the present time, I have a pessimistic view about the future of psychodynamic psychotherapy as a discipline. Many changes are taking place in the world at large, and in medicine in particular, that do not bode well for the future of psychotherapy. I will first discuss the situation in the society at large, then in medicine, then in psychiatry, and finally the implications of these changes for child and adolescent psychotherapists in other disciplines.

The Ever-Burgeoning Psychopathy
in American Society

I believe that American society (in common with many other societies) has become increasingly psychopathic in the last 15 to 20 years. This is not only reflected by increasing rates of homicide, rape, arson, and theft, but by more subtle manifestations of self-serving behavior on the part of people in general. Its manifestations are ubiquitous. Children are being sexually abused with increasing frequency, not only by their parents but by their teachers, scout masters, clergymen, and others who have access to them. Anyone willing to pay $25,000 can get a forged medical degree with associated counterfeit credentials. There was a time when London policeman did not carry guns because even the lowest criminals could be relied upon to refrain from shooting an unarmed person. This is no longer the case. With increasing frequency scientists in academic life are submitting falsified data in order to enhance their reputations and chances for promotion. The U.S. government is facing increasing difficulties getting repayment for student loans. In New York City, census collectors in 1980 were filmed sitting in or standing around their cars filling out batches of census forms while listening to rock music. In the same city construction inspectors have refused to accept promotions because they will then be removed from the more lucrative payoffs to be gained on the street. I could continue and I am sure the reader can supply his or her own examples of the increasing psychopathy of our society.

Payment of Fees

When I was in medical school, a physician who required patients to pay their fees at the time services were rendered would have been considered materialistic, "money hungry," and "grub-by." Bills were sent and it was expected that the vast majority of patients in treatment would have a sense of responsibility with regard to their payments. Any physician now who trusts most patients to pay for services in the future is not going to remain in practice very long. Most physicians now unabashedly and unashamedly request that their patients pay at the time services are rendered. In fact, there are many physicians who will not admit a patient to the hospital unless payment is made in advance. And many hospitals (especially private hospitals) utilize the same procedure. This change may not affect significantly practice in other branches of medicine, but it can compromise psychiatric treatment. Implicit in the demand that payment be made at the time services are rendered is the notion of distrust. There is no way to separate the two. The patient is basically being told: "I want you to pay *now*, because I don't trust you to pay me in *the future*." Increasingly, psychiatrists are coming to appreciate that the traditional monthly bill is becoming an anachronism, applicable in simpler times, but no longer consistent with survival in the more cutthroat world of the late 20th century.

At this point I still allow my adult patients to pay me at the end of each month. I take the position that it is better to lose a certain percentage of my billings than to say uniformly to all adult patients that I distrust them. If, however, a patient begins to renege, I am quick to bring this up in treatment and to provide therapeutic justification for more frequent payments or even payment every session. In this situation, distrust cannot be viewed as an inappropriate generalization in which an innocent party is being distrusted because others act in a distrustful way. Rather, my distrust of the patient stems from untrustworthy behavior exhibited by him or her. With my child and adolescent patients, however, I ask the parents to pay at the time of each session. I am not completely happy with this practice, but it is better than the traditional method because of the high parental default rate I was experiencing in recent years. The default rate of childrens' parents was higher than that of adult patients because there was less direct monitoring and surveillance of the parents. Unfortunate as it is, that is the reality of the situation. This practice has not affected my relationship with my child and adolescent patients because it is not *they* I am distrusting, but their parents. One could argue here that I am compromising my relationship with parents and, therefore, as one who has spoken so much about the importance of the therapist's relationship with parents, I am compromising indirectly my child and adolescent patients' treatment. I admit to this compromise. My only answer is that I too have to earn a living.

Malpractice Suits

The everburgeoning rate of malpractice suits has also had its effect on medicine. At the time of this writing there are neurosurgeons in the greater New York City area who pay a malpractice insurance premium of $105,000 per year. And there are neurosurgeons in Florida who pay over $225,000 per year. Although these figures are almost unimaginable, they are true. Young people cannot enter a field in which they have to pay such astronomical premiums starting on the first day they open their offices. Judicious physicians practice what has come to be called "defensive medicine." Here, they must always be thinking about the potential malpractice suit that may be brought in the course of conducting day-to-day medical practice. Tests are ordered which would not previously have been requested because of the remote possibility that the physicians might be accused of being sloppy or negligent. The chances of the test's being positive may be one in 100,000, but the spectre of being cross-examined on a witness stand because of the failure to have ordered a particular test results in this extra expense to the patient. It appears that there are no longer any such things as naturally occurring birth defects. If a child is born with a congenital anomaly, the parents see nothing inappropriate about suing the obstetrician. The situation has gotten so bad that many OB-GYN practitioners have stopped delivering babies entirely and confine themselves soley to gynecological practice. There are thousands of parents of children with neurologically based learning disabilities who are suing obstetricians. The child may have nothing more wrong with him or her than the fact that the IQ is at the 20th percentile level. Accordingly, a normal variation is given a diagnostic label—a disease—and an innocent obstetrician is then sued for malpractice. And schools are being sued for not having brought such children up to normal levels of intellectual functioning. Psychiatrists practice with the fear that their reports will be used as evidence in malpractice litigation. Accordingly, they are becoming increasingly cautious about what they say in their reports, and the result is that these are becoming progressively less useful.

I believe that we in medicine should certainly be accountable for our errors and that we should not be immune from malpractice suits. However, we have a malpractice situation here in the United

States that is unconscionable. At the present time, the ratio of one lawyer for 800 people in the population is actually increasing. There are many hungry lawyers and many doctors who are viewed as being "rich." (Remember the bumper sticker: "Become a doctor and support a lawyer.") Furthermore, we have the despicable practice of the contingency arrangement. Under this program a patient need not put down a cent to institute malpractice litigation. The attorney works for nothing in the hope that he or she will win and thereby receive anywhere from 33 to 50 percent of the award. Most countries in the world consider this an unsavory practice and it is outlawed. But it cannot be so easily outlawed in the United States because the state legislatures are largely populated by attorneys, the friends and relatives of the malpractice lawyers. The malpractice situation is another example of the general psychopathy of our society—the psychopathy that is compromising the clinical practice of psychiatry.

The Craze for Quick Cures

Another manifestation of the psychopathy in our society that is affecting psychiatric practice is the desire for quick solutions and rapid cures. I believe that the vast majority of patients who interrupt treatment prematurely do so because they are dissatisfied with a therapeutic program that involves effort over a long period. Psychodynamic therapies of the kinds described in this book generally take time, and sometimes a long time. The factors that have contributed to the development of the youngster's symptoms may have been generations in the making. The patient may have been exposed to the detrimental environmental influences from the day of birth. It is unreasonable to expect the therapist to undo all these contributing factors in a short period. Yet, most patients and parents want just that. And, as the old law of supply and demand dictates, when people are willing to pay for the things they are demanding, there will be people who will supply what is being demanded and accept payment for their services. It matters little whether the product being supplied is of any value. What matters primarily is whether people are willing to pay money for it.

Accordingly, there is an ever-burgeoning supply of practitioners who promise quick solutions. The most influential of these in the field of psychiatry are the so-called "biological psychiatrists." Although there is a wide range of opinions regarding the role of nature vs. nurture among people who espouse this position, their general view is that nature (genes, constitution, metabolic process- es, etc.) is the primary determinant of psychiatric disorder. Theirs is certainly an attractive position. Rather than spend long periods going into background history, rather than undergo the tedious process of trying to understand underlying psychodynamics, all one has to do is provide a medicine that presumably will correct the biological abnormality that is theorized to be the cause of the disorder. When it comes to asking for grants, these people are obviously at an advantage over those of us who want to investigate the longer and presumably less predictably successful kinds of treatment. Those who fund such research (whether it be the government or other institutions) are more likely to be attracted to these presumably more "cost-effective" forms of treatment.

A parallel situation exists in psychology. Psychodynamically oriented psychologists, who believe that prolonged and intensive psychotherapies are likely to be the most efficacious, are not being viewed benevolently by those who provide money for research, training, and teaching. Rather, behavior therapists who believe that inquiry into the unconscious is a waste of time and money are more likely to obtain grants. They are more attractive, as well, to schools and institutions, where large numbers of patients are provided services. There was a time when we spoke of doctors providing treatment to patients. Now the lingo calls us "providers" and our treatment "delivery of services." The word *delivery* connotes to me someone in a truck delivering a product. We have not reached that point yet, but I would not be surprised if very soon we start referring to our patients as "the customers."

**Training in Child and
Adolescent Psychiatry**

As a result of this situation there has been a dramatic shift in the type of training young psychiatrists now receive. Most of the medical school training programs in the United States began in the

1940s and 1950s when psychoanalytic theory reigned supreme. During that period there was hardly a department that was not chaired by a classically oriented psychoanalyst. In the late 1960s and early 1970s the pendulum began to shift in favor of the biological psychiatrists. This occurred at a time when hospitals became increasingly pressured to support ever more complex and sophisticated forms of medical treatment. Furthermore, hospitals could no longer rely on the relatively inexpensive services provided by professionals such as nurses, attendants, laboratory technicians, etc. People could no longer be relied upon to dedicate themselves to the treatment of the ill with little financial remuneration. On the one hand, one could say that the shrinkage of such dedicated individuals was related to a psychopathic society in which fewer individuals were willing to make sacrifices in compliance with noble principles such as self-sacrifice, sympathy for the underprivileged, and dedication to the needs of the poor. On the other hand, one could argue that people decided that they no longer wanted to be exploited by hospital administrators. I believe that both factors operated here with the net result that there are now fewer people who are working in hospitals because of high and noble principles, and there are also fewer people who are being exploited. Unions became stronger, wage demands more stringent, and hospitals had to cut back in every possible way to survive. They became increasingly dependent on their outside funding.

Up to the 1970s a departmental chairperson (there were mainly chair*men* in those days) was chosen primarily on the basis of medical expertise and dedication, and only secondarily on administrative capabilities and funding sources. Hospitals now find themselves in the position of having to use the latter criteria for selection much more than the former. We are living at a time when a person who is a candidate for a departmental chair is judged primarily on his or her "track record" in acquiring funding; medical expertise is of only secondary consideration. The effect of this on psychiatry has been to place psychodynamically oriented people at a tremendous disadvantage with regard to chairing departments. This has reached a point where there is hardly a psychiatry department in the United States today that is chaired by a dynamically oriented psychiatrist. As is to be expected, the chairpersons themselves not only hire people who think the way they do but also favor individuals who themselves have good "track records" regarding funding for their work.

As a result of this situation, the young psychiatrist in training may have little if any psychodynamically oriented therapeutic experience. In many of these departments the primary therapeutic modalities are determined by what is short, seemingly quick, and "cost effective." Drug therapy, obviously, satisfies this proviso. To a lesser extent, behavior modification is attractive for the same reasons. Cognitive therapies, whose primary aim is to change distorted thinking relatively quickly, are also very much in vogue. Many people in these programs see no need to get background history about the patient's family or to investigate into underlying psychodynamics. The symptom is viewed as the disease and symptom alleviation or removal is considered the only goal of treatment. Even the manual of psychiatric diagnoses (*DSM-IV*) reflects this philosophy. It is basically antipsychodynamic. The selection of a disorder's name is based primarily, if not exclusively, on the manifest symptoms.

One of the most unfortunate outcomes of all this is the diagnostic category known as *attention deficit disorder* (ADD). If one looks at the charts of child patients in hospitals, clinics, and the offices of child psychiatrists, child neurologists, pediatricians, child psychologists, and school guidance counselors, the "disease" is indeed epidemic. It has become the rubber-stamp diagnosis of the 1980s. Any child who does not listen to his or her parents or teachers is quickly labeled "ADD." If one is to believe these reports, we are experiencing an epidemic greater than we ever had with any other disorder known to medicine.

The implication is that these children are suffering with a neurophysiological derangement which may or may not be associated with hyperactivity (also presumed to be neurophysiologic in etiology). With this assumption, the next step is to provide a convenient drug: enter psychostimulant medication. At this time it is reasonable to say that psychostimulant medication is being prescribed by the ton—literally by the ton. All this is quick and slick, but a terrible disservice to patients. I believe that the vast majority of children who are diagnosed as having ADD have problems that have nothing to do with their attentional capacity, but more to do with psychogenic rather than neurophysiological factors (Gardner,

1996). Their difficulties, I believe, are more readily explained by family and other environmental influences. Most children who are considered to have ADD are diagnosed on an observational or even hearsay basis. When objective criteria for attentional capacity are utilized (such as the Digit Span, Arithmetic, and Coding subtests of the *WISC-R*) the diagnosis cannot be justified.

Elsewhere (1987b) I discuss in detail my own studies that support my position that the ADD label (not the hyperactivity label) is a myth that exists in the brains of those who make the diagnosis and not in the brains of those who are being so diagnosed. I do believe, however, that *some* hyperactive children are indeed so on a neurophysiological basis and *will* be helped by psychostimulant medication. My main point here is that the popularity of the ADD and hyperactivity labels and the ubiquitous use of psychostimulant medication is another manifestation of the search for quick and simple cures for complicated problems, the worship of cost-effectiveness, the anxieties engendered by introspective psychotherapeutic approaches, the prevailing psychopathy of our society, and the resulting dehumanization of psychiatry.

Prepaid Treatment Plans

Another phenomenon that has compromised significantly the quality of psychiatric care, and threatens to do so even more in the immediate future, is the increasing popularity of prepaid treatment plans. Their main purpose has been to provide patients with lower cost treatment. One can argue that the present medical system leaves much to be desired. Rich patients clearly receive far better care than the poor. They have the opportunity to select their doctors freely and have the wherewithal to pay their fees, no matter how high. On the other end of the scale, the indigent generally attend hospital clinics, have no choice of physicians, and are often treated by those in training. As is usually the case, those in the middle class get something in between. Prepaid insurance plans provide such care, especially for the middle class. There is no question that many physicians have exploited the public with their unconscionable fees. If a person has a brain tumor and all the neurosurgeons in private practice are charging $15,000 for its removal, the patient has little choice but to pay. There is no question that this is a form of exploitation. There is no question that some kind of backlash was predictable. There is no question also that people in clinics have been getting inadequate treatment and that some kind of retaliatory reaction was also foreseeable. However, indigents are less likely to involve themselves effectively in movements for their rights than those who are better educated and in a better financial position. Some of the prepaid plans are manifestations of this backlash. I discuss here some of the most well known, those that do not provide free choice of physician within the plan.

In recent years we have witnessed the establishment of *health maintenance organizations* (HMOs). Many large companies have traditionally provided their workers with the opportunity to select their physicians. Under a typical program the worker would be reimbursed a significant percentage of the cost of medical care. The basic philosophy was that an individual should be free to choose any physician he or she wished to, without any external restrictions. In recent years companies have found that it is more "cost-effective" to engage the services of, and even to build their own, clinics and hospitals and to give their workers a choice. If one chooses the company's medical facilities, one may pay nothing or very little. One is still free to obtain treatment from an outside physician, but one will get little if any reimbursement for doing so. Obviously, under such a program, very few people are going to select the latter course. Large companies have not only set up their own clinics but even their own hospitals. Those who have not set up their own have contracted with private hospitals that were established for this purpose. Insurance companies, as well, have found it an attractive program. The physicians in these organizations are often employees. They are paid specific salaries and their work is monitored, again with regard to whether or not it is "cost-effective." One result of this trend has been a progressive shrinkage of private practice. Young physicians today cannot generally look forward to the autonomy of individual practice because an increasing percentage of their potential patient population is now receiving care from HMOs. They too must become salaried employees if they are to make a living in the field of medicine.

There are four specialities in medicine that have been particularly hurt by HMOs, specifically dermatology, allergy, plastic surgery, and psychiatry. The consensus among administrators of HMOs is that these specialities often provide frivolous treatment and the therapy is frequently prolonged unnecessarily for the financial benefit of the physician. Accordingly, the funds allotted for treatment in these four categories is generally a much smaller fraction of the traditional than in other medical specialties. Although one might argue that much of the "bread and butter" of plastic surgery is unnecessary cosmetic surgery, one cannot as easily give a convincing argument that much of psychiatric therapy is equally frivolous. The result, however, is that physicians and patients under HMO plans are told that they must accomplish their treatment in a fixed number of sessions. Therapists who claim that therapy takes much longer are not likely to remain employed very long. Those who subscribe to a theory that short-term therapy is as good as the long-term variation will be viewed with favor. This is a ripoff on the public. As mentioned so frequently throughout this book, psychotherapy can only be meaningful in the context of an ongoing relationship, and one cannot put a fixed number of hours on the development, evolution, and therapeutic benefit of this relationship. And the next step has already taken place. Therapists in private practice, suffering from the emigration of their patient population to HMOs, are now taking jobs in HMOs. And they are going along with the philosophy that treatment can indeed be accomplished in a predetermined number of sessions.

A related development is the establishment of *preferred-provider organizations* (PPOs). Here, private practitioners, in an attempt to compete with HMOs for patients, group together and bid for service contracts with insurance companies, industries, etc. These organizations do comparative shopping in the medical marketplace and contract with a group of providers who agree on a predetermined list of charges. These practitioners, then, are charging higher rates to patients who are not members of these plans than they are to subscribers. Again, it is unreasonable to assume that patients who are receiving care at the lower fee are going to get the same quality of care and attention as those who are paying more. And this is especially the case in psychiatric treatment where the fixed charges are likely to limit the number of sessions available to the patient.

Another arrangement is the *independent practice association* (IPA). IPAs were also established to compete with HMOs for patients. Here, a group of physicians gets together and forms its own service plan. Whereas in HMOs and PPOs an outside organization, such as an industry or an insurance company, sets up the plan, in the IPA the doctors themselves organize and administer the program. They therefore save the costs of paying outside administrators. As is true for PPOs, doctors seeing patients under the IPA plan generally charge two fees, a higher fee for their genuinely private patients and a lower fee for those who come under the service contract. Again, I have the same reservations about IPAs as I do about HMOs and PPOs, namely, that psychiatric care has got to be compromised by the limited amount of time available under these fixed service plans.

Another development that is compromising significantly the quality of care in the field of psychiatry is the growth of the *diagnostic related groups* (DRGs). Again, in order to improve the cost-effectiveness of medical care and to increase the efficiency of such treatment (especially with regard to paperwork), many of the payers of medical care (insurance companies, Blue Cross/Blue Shield, Medicare, Medicaid, etc) have made up a list of hundreds of disorders for which hospitals provide treatment. The hospital is given a fixed amount of money for the treatment of patients suffering with one or more of these disorders—regardless of the number of days in the hospital and regardless of the kinds of medicines, procedures, operations, etc. that are required. The amount of payment is based on the average cost for the treatment of the particular condition in the recent past. Although this approach certainly saves much paperwork and perhaps even reduces the number of days a patient will remain in the hospital, it cannot but compromise psychiatric treatment. It behooves hospitals to discharge patients at the earliest possible time, and this is likely to result in patients' not being allowed to stay the optimum amount of time. Doctors who keep their patients in longer than the average may find that their treatment is becoming "cost ineffective." They will be advised by hospital administrators to shorten the duration of their patients' stays or risk the displeasure of those who pay their salaries and/or determine their suitability for enjoying the benefits of hospital privileges.

I consider all of these prepayment plans to pose the risk of curtailed treatment for patients. To me plans like these, when applied to psychiatry, can be compared to restricting marriages to 7.3 years, because that is the average duration of the marriages in the community in which the couple is marrying. The analogy is applicable because the therapeutic relationship, if a good one, has similarities to the good marriage with regard to the intimacy and closeness that emerges. The other drawback of these prepaid plans is that physicians on salary are not as likely to work as enthusiastically and with as high motivation as those who enjoy the promise of higher earnings for enhanced competence and the establishment for themselves of a reputation for excellence. Most human beings (including doctors) are not so saint-like that they will work as assiduously for a fixed income as they will in a situation where there is the promise of greater rewards. In some ideal world of perfect people, such differentiations may not be made. In our real world, however, real doctors are not going to give as much attention and commitment to their prepaid patients as they will to those who provide promise of greater remuneration. And this difference is especially true in psychiatry when one compares the remuneration for a few sessions under a fixed-fee program and that which is possible from a private patient in an ongoing therapeutic program.

The Dehumanization of Psychiatric Care

If the reader detects a note of pessimism in the above, he or she is correct. I have little reason to feel confident about the future of the field of child and adolescent psychiatry, whether practiced in the hospital, clinic, or private setting. Hospitals and clinics are training automatons who provide a dehumanized kind of treatment. In recent years I am seeing with increasing frequency reports that are completely devoid of information about family background, developmental history, and underlying psychodynamics. The patients are "processed" and the care "delivered." The clinic administrators pride themselves on the total number of people they can "process" in a given period and gloat over comparisons between their own turnover rates and those of previous administrators, who worked when traditional psychotherapeutic techniques were being utilized. Patients come to the clinic and, while waiting to see their doctors, fill out symptom checklists. These are then fed into a computer and compared with previous symptom checklists. By the time the patient is seen, the therapist has the up-to-date data in hand and is allegedly in a position to assess the patient's "progress." The whole session may take five to ten minutes, during which time the primary purpose is to adjust medication and write prescriptions. There is little if any time for any discussion of the human problems that may be contributing significantly to the patient's problems. But even if there were, the doctor has not been trained adequately in psychodynamic therapy and may have little if any conviction for it.

The young physician who is thinking of entering the field of psychiatry and who recognizes how unconscionable the system is, has great difficulty finding training in a more humane setting. If the physician were to find more humanistic therapy being provided in a nonmedical training program, such as psychology for example, he or she would still be faced with formidable problems. Certainly, such training would not be recognized toward certification in a medical specialty and psychologists might not even recognize the physician's training as being adequate for admission to the program. If the individual decided to go through one of the dehumanized medical programs and tolerate its deficiencies in the hope of rectifying them later, he or she will have had little training to serve as a basis for the subsequent more humane type of psychiatric treatment.

Those who recognize how unconscionably inadequate are our present training programs in psychiatry have little place to turn. When young people ask my advice about where in psychiatry they can train, I tell them I know of no center within the field of medicine. I suspect that there may be a few programs in which psychodynamically oriented therapy is still the prevailing approach. However, I have no optimism that such programs will remain long in effect. In every program that I am familiar with, the process has been the same: a psychodynamically oriented chairperson has been replaced by someone with a deep commitment to the biological approach. Dynamically oriented chairpersons have been fired, prematurely retired, eased out, forced out, or thrown out! In short, what we are witnessing is the corruption of a field by lust for money. The aforementioned influences that are eroding the field at a frighteningly rapid rate are formidable, and I see little evidence that things will change in the near future.

CHILD AND ADOLESCENT
PSYCHOTHERAPY IN NONMEDICAL
DISCIPLINES

Now to other disciplines that are providing psychotherapy. There was a time, less than ten years ago, when psychologists were warring with psychiatrists with regard to who has the right to do psychotherapy. That war is over. There was no truce; there was no armistice. Rather, psychiatry just walked away from the battlefield. Psychiatry views itself as having "returned to medicine." The recent attitude of psychiatry has been: "Leave psychotherapy to the psychologist and the social workers, they can hold the hands of people who need that sort of thing." The general public has similarly come to view psychiatrists almost exclusively as the purveyors of drugs and as therapists for psychotics, severe depressives, and others who have physical disorders that require shock therapy and/or medication. Psychologists are now viewed by the general public as the providers of psychotherapy. This may be a good thing considering the deplorable state of present-day medical residency programs. But it is now the psychologists who are fighting with the social workers over who should have the right to do psychotherapy. And others have quickly entered the arena: pastoral counselors, nurse practitioners, family counselors, marital counselors, and a large assortment of others with varying degrees of training and expertise. There is likely to be a Pyrrhic victory in the end because if these people are fighting over patients for private practice, as the HMOs, PPOs, and IPAs continue to grow there will be very few patients left, if any. They will end up finding that what they have "won" will be jobs that will confine them to "cost-effective" therapeutic programs with a specific number of hours allotted to each patient.

FINAL COMMENTS

It would be an error for the reader to concude that I am white-washing completely psychodynamic psychotherapy in this section of my book. Biological psychiatry, in part, enjoyed popularity as a justifiable backlash against the widespread enthusiasm for classical psychoanalysis and its derivative techniques. There was a grandiosity to some of these practitioners that bordered on the delusional. They considered themselves to have had in the palm of their hands the definitive and the most effective form of psychotherapeutic treatment ever devised in the history of humankind. Those who disagreed with them were viewed as having psychological problems that had not been properly analyzed. Furthermore, the length of the treatment programs they were utilizing was inordinately long, even if there was the funding available for such prolonged treatment. The idea that most patients be treated four or five times a week was patently absurd.

And there are those who were (and still are) providing worthless treatment that is referred to as "play therapy." I have come across numerous child therapists who actually believe that play therapy is nothing more than playing with a child. They have little if any insight into the fact that the play, if it is to justifiably warrant the name *play therapy*, must be more therapy than play and that the play should only be a vehicle for the transmission of therapeutic messages and experiences. These practitioners also may have contributed to the backlash as it has been applied to child therapy. Hundreds of thousands of hours have been wasted while therapists have been taking children to soda fountains, baseball games, circuses, etc. under the aegis of child therapy. And many of these concepts are held by those who work with adolescents—especially younger ones.

So there was much housecleaning that had to be done (and still has to be done) among those who do child and adolescent therapy. I recognize that this is an extremely pessimistic note on which to end a book. However, it is the reality of the world in which we are living and to deny it would be foolish and self-destructive. If all that I predict here regarding psychodynamic psychotherapy comes to pass (and much of it has already happened), then a book like this might not prove very useful—because very few people will be in a position to provide the kind of therapy described herein. I have recognized this while writing this series but still felt that it had to be written. I felt that I had to write a compendium of my contributions and pull together my ideas. There are still enough people at this point who have the autonomy and flexibility to practice the kind of psychodynamic therapy described in it. Perhaps one day there will be some kind of backlash against the recent depravities, and more people will come to appreciate how unconscionable many present therapeutic programs are. My hope is that they will work toward bringing us once again into an atmosphere in which more humane therapeutic approaches will prevail. Perhaps this entire series of three books may serve (admittedly in a small way) to inspire others like myself who are still striving to maintain what was good in the past and to contribute to its reflowering in the future.

REFERENCES

Aichorn, A. (1925). *Wayward Youth.* New York: World Publishing Co., 1954.

Christ, J. (1974). Outpatient treatment of adolescents and their families. In *American Handbook of Psychiatry, Vol. II,* ed. G. Caplan, pp. 339–352. New York: Basic Books.

Gardner, R. A. (1973). *The Talking, Feeling, and Doing Game.* Cresskill, NJ: Creative Therapeutics.

——— (1979). *The Objective Diagnosis of Minimal Brain Dysfunction.* Cresskill, NJ: Creative Therapeutics.

——— (1983). *The Boys and Girls' Book About One-Parent Families.* Cresskill, NJ: Creative Therapeutics.

——— (1986). *Child Custody Litigation: A Guide for Parents and Mental Health Professionals.* Cresskill, NJ: Creative Therapeutics.

——— (1987a). *The Parental Alienation Syndrome and the Differentiation between Fabricated and Genuine Child Sex Abuse.* Cresskill, NJ: Creative Therapeutics.

——— (1987b). *Hyperactivity, the So-Called Attention Deficit Disorder, and the Group of MBD Syndromes.* Cresskill, NJ: Creative Therapeutics.

——— (1996). *Psychogenic Learning Disabilities: Psychodyanamics and Psychotherapy.* Cresskill, NJ: Creative Therapeutics.

———— (1999a). *Developmental Conflicts and Diagnostic Evaluation in Adolescent Psychotherapy.* Northvale, NJ: Jason Aronson.

———— (1999b). *Individual and Group Therapy and Work with Parents in Adolescent Psychotherapy.* Northvale, NJ: Jason Aronson.

Gardner, R. A., Gardner, A. K., Caemmerer, A., and Broman, M. (1979). An instrument for measuring hyperactivity and other signs of minimal brain dysfunction. *Journal of Clinical Child Psychology* 8(3):173–179.

Gittelman-Klein, R. (1975). Pharmacotherapy and management of pathological separation anxiety. *International Journal of Mental Health* 4:255–270.

Gittelman-Klein, R., and Klein, D. F. (1973). School phobia: diagnostic considerations in the light of imipramine effects. *Journal of Nervous and Mental Diseases* 156:199–215.

Holmes, D. J. (1964). *The Adolescent in Psychotherapy.* Boston: Little, Brown.

Johnson, A. M. (1949). Sanctions for superego lacunae of adolescents. In *Searchlights on Delinquency,* ed. K. R. Eissler, pp. 225–245. New York: International Universities Press.

Johnson, A. M., and Szurek, S. A. (1952). The genesis of antisocial acting out in children and adults. *Psychoanalytic Quarterly* 21:323–343.

Klein, M. (1932). *The Psychoanalysis of Children.* London: Hogarth.

Lieberman, L. K. (1981). *The Litigious Society.* New York: Basic Books.

Marshall, R. J. (1979). Antisocial youth. In *Basic Handbook of Child Psychiatry, Vol. III,* ed. S. I. Harrison, pp. 536–554. New York: Basic Books.

———— (1983). A psychoanalytic perspective on the diagnosis and development of juvenile delinquents. In *Personality Theory, Moral Development and Criminal Behavior,* ed. W. S. Laufer and J. M. Day, pp. 119–144. Lexington, MA: D. C. Heath.

Rinsley, D. B. (1974). Residential treatment of adolescents. In *American Handbook of Psychiatry,* ed. G. Caplan, vol II, pp. 353–366. New York: Basic Books.

Sarason, I. G., and Sarason, B. R. (1980). *Abnormal Psychology* 3rd ed. Englewood Cliffs, NJ: Prentice–Hall.

Schimel, J. S. (1974). Problems of delinquency and their treatment. In *American Handbook of Psychiatry,* ed G. Caplan, vol II, pp. 264–274. New York: Basic Books.

Simmons, K. (1987a). Adolescent suicide: second leading death cause. *Journal of the American Medical Association* 257(24):3329–3330.

———— (1987b). Task force to make recommendations for adolescents in terms of suicide risk. *Journal of the American Medical Association* 257(24):3330–3332.

Stone, L. A. (1979). Residential treatment. In *Basic Handbook of Child Psychiatry,* ed. S. I. Harrison, vol. III, pp. 231–262. New York: Basic Books.

Toolan, J. M. (1974). Depression and suicide. In *American Handbook of Psychiatry,* ed. G. Caplan, vol. II, pp. 294–306. New York: Basic Books.

Wensley, S. (1987). Portrait of adolescent suicide. In *P&S (Columbia University, College of Physicians and Surgeons)* 7(2):14–17.

Westman, J. C. (1979). Psychiatric day treatment. In *Basic Handbook of Child Psychiatry, Vol. III,* ed. S. I. Harrison, pp. 288–299. New York: Basic Books.

Zinn, D. (1979). Hospital treatment of the adolescent. In *Basic Handbook of Child Psychiatry, Vol. III,* ed S. I. Harrison, pp. 263–288. New York: Basic Books.

AUTHOR INDEX

SUBJECT INDEX